SpringerBriefs in Psychology

Advances in Child and Family Policy and Practice

Editor in chief

More information about this series at http://www.springer.com/series/10143

Mary E. Haskett
Editor

Child and Family Well-Being and Homelessness

Integrating Research into Practice and Policy

Springer

Editor
Mary E. Haskett
Department of Psychology
North Carolina State University
Raleigh, NC, USA

ISSN 2192-8363 ISSN 2192-8371 (electronic)
SpringerBriefs in Psychology
ISBN 978-3-319-50885-6 ISBN 978-3-319-50886-3 (eBook)
DOI 10.1007/978-3-319-50886-3

Library of Congress Control Number: 2017931313

Printed on acid-free paper

This Springer imprint is published by Springer Nature
The registered company is Springer International Publishing AG
The registered company address is: Gewerbestrasse 11, 6330 Cham, Switzerland

Executive Summary: Enhancing Public Policy to Promote Well-Being of Parents and Children Experiencing Homelessness

This summary of policy recommendations focuses on three areas: (1) the integration of policies and practices for families experiencing homelessness; (2) the promotion of healthy families; and (3) building the evidence base to guide effective policy. This is not an exhaustive list; rather, these recommendations are drawn from results of the innovative studies in this monograph of *Advances in Child and Family Policy and Practice*. Broader policy recommendations are available from the National Association for the Education of Homeless Children and Youth, the National Alliance to End Homelessness, the Bassuk Center on Homeless and Vulnerable Children & Youth, The U.S. DHHS Administration for Children and Families (see especially the new Policy Statement on Meeting the Needs of Families with Young Children Experiencing and At Risk of Homelessness), and the U.S. Interagency Council on Homelessness.

Integrate Policies and Practices

- **Require and Support Coordinated Policies Across Sectors**. *Policies and funding sources must be linked more closely* across agencies that serve homeless children and families. To illustrate, the National Center on Early Head Start-Child Care Partnerships (jointly funded by the Office of Head Start and the Office of Child Care) encourages development of *formal partnerships* between Early Head Start and child care programs. Partnerships should expand to include McKinney-Vento Coordinators for Education of Homeless Children and Youths, IDEA Part C (Early Intervention) programs, and CCDF services. Funding should be allocated for technical assistance for implementing and sustaining the coordinated policies.
- **Integrate Coordinated Cross-System Support Services with Housing Support**. Availability of affordable housing and sufficient federal and state funding for housing vouchers for all eligible families are essential for ending

family homelessness, but there is also a critical role for *psychosocial services* in stabilization of vulnerable families. The Bassuk Center's Services Matter report (www.bassukcenter.org) delineates eight essential components of a comprehensive two-generational response to family homelessness that involves coordinating delivery of services to support the entire family.

Promote Healthy Families

- **Mandate Use of Two-Generational Family-Centered Assessment Processes.** Families without homes are a heterogeneous group, though they share common risk factors. Given variability across families, a *comprehensive screening and assessment process* is vital to identify needs of all family members and reduce wasteful "one-size-fits-all" approaches.
- **Increase Access to Early Care and Education.** Given the disproportionate number of families with very young children who are homeless and the many barriers faced by families seeking care for their children, there is a clear and compelling need for increased *access to high-quality early care and education* for these families. Provisions in the reauthorized Child Care Development Block Grant (CCDBG) have incorporated McKinney-Vento concepts into the policies of the Individuals with Disabilities Education Act (IDEA) and Head Start. Pending adequate funding, the CCDBG may provide additional resources to homeless services providers to help their clients access early childhood resources. Further, the Improving Head Start for School Readiness Act of 2007 mandated the prioritization of children experiencing homelessness; unfortunately, waitlists persist, so *adequate appropriation of funds* must follow mandates.
- **Prioritize Parenting Resources to Families Experiencing Homelessness.** Positive parenting promotes resilience of children who face the loss of their home. Like all parents, those experiencing homelessness are eager to receive parenting support. In the face of enormous stress and adversity, parents experiencing homelessness require *greater access to parenting support.* Prioritizing families without homes for federally funded programs such as those supported by the Maternal, Infant, and Early Childhood Home Visiting (MIECHV) program, as well as Early Head Start and Head Start programs, could promote positive parenting and reduce early social-emotional-behavioral challenges of young homeless children and prevent later mental health problems.

Build the Evidence Base to Guide Effective Policy

- **Improve Data Collection and Fund Research on Family Homelessness.** Effective policies to end family homelessness must be driven by high-quality data. In the absence of consistent and comprehensive data, policies are ill informed at best or ineffective at worst. Currently, the evidence base for effective housing and services to address family homelessness is not well developed. The pace of knowledge development must accelerate at a pace that reflects the rapidly growing number of homeless families and the complex nature of their needs. Improved data collection on parent and child functioning and services delivered by individual programs (IDEA Part C, CCDF, etc.) and through HUD's Homeless Management Information Systems (HMIS) would provide critical information to develop appropriate policy responses.
- **Shape Research Funding.** In addition to enhancing existing data collection systems, public and private research grants should be made available at higher levels for investigations of family homelessness, specifically in the following areas:

  (a) Fund research to examine implementation and effects of *evidence-based programs* delivered in housing programs to promote positive parenting and reduce risk for child maltreatment and to treat parent and child mental health challenges. Studies should be funded at a level that will ensure they are sufficiently powered to determine not only what works but also for whom the intervention works, under what conditions the intervention is effective, and when and at what dosage it should be delivered.

  (b) Develop and replicate innovative systems changes, including *models of collaboration* as recommended by experts and as described in this Brief. Investigations are needed to identify factors that (a) promote such collaboration, (b) ensure consistency, fidelity, and sustainability of collaborative models, and (c) facilitate capacity for scaling the models. The relatively new area of implementation science can inform these investigations.

  (c) Fund investigations in resilience science to gain a greater *understanding of the sources of resilience* that enable some vulnerable children and families without homes to adjust and even thrive. These studies should be designed to assess predictors of parent and child functioning over time, from the time they experience their first episode of housing instability through the process of obtaining permanent living situations.

  (d) Fund pilot programs to develop evidence-based *methods to improve early childhood outcomes* for vulnerable young children who are homeless and unstably housed. Early childhood is a critical developmental period; failure to fully support the developmental needs of infants, toddlers, and preschoolers without homes is unacceptable. For example, funding is needed to ascertain effects on child outcomes of new tools such as the Early Childhood Self-Assessment Tool for Emergency Shelters developed by the USDHHS Administration for Children and Families.

Conclusion

Family homelessness must be addressed by a comprehensive, integrated set of policy and practice strategies and public and private funding for a purposeful research agenda to build the evidence base. Family's needs must be at the center of decision-making and policy-building. Solutions are within reach, but greater political and public commitment is critical to reduce homelessness and aid parents without homes in advancing their lives and supporting their children's futures.

Contents

About the Editor

Mary E. Haskett, Ph.D., is Professor of Psychology at North Carolina State University, where her research focuses on factors that shape parenting, the influences of parenting on children's social-emotional development, adjustment of children with a history of maltreatment, and understanding approaches to support parents and children experiencing homelessness. She and her graduate students currently conduct research on interventions to promote positive parenting among parents residing in emergency shelters and transitional housing. Dr. Haskett co-edited (with S. Perlman and B.A. Cowan) a leading text on family homelessness, *Supporting Families Experiencing Homelessness: Current Practices and Future Directions* (Springer, 2014). She received the 2016 National Association for the Education of Homeless Children and Youth, Dr. Staci Perlman Achievements in Research Award.

Contributors

Amanda Albu Office of Institutional Research and Assessment, Temple University, USA

Gerald J. August Department of Family Social Science, University of Minnesota, St. Paul, MN, USA

Ellen L. Bassuk Center for Social Innovation, Needham Heights, MA, USA

Carie Bires Ounce of Prevention, Chicago, IL, USA

Preston A. Britner Department of Human Development and Family Studies, University of Connecticut, Storrs, CT, USA

J.J. Cutuli Department of Psychology, Rutgers University—Camden, Camden, NJ, USA

Carmela J. DeCandia Licensed Psychologist and Organizational Consultant, Newton, MA, USA

Anne F. Farrell Chapin Hall at the University of Chicago, Chicago, IL, USA

Abigail H. Gewirtz Department of Family Social Science and Institute of Child Development, University of Minnesota, St. Paul, MN, USA

Mary E. Haskett Department of Psychology, North Carolina State University, Raleigh, NC, USA

Janette E. Herbers Department of Psychology, Villanova University, Villanova, PA, USA

Kendal Holtrop Department of Family and Child Sciences, Florida State University, Tallahassee, FL, USA

Charles H. Kieffer The Cloudburst Group, Landover, MD, USA

Lyuboslava Kolarova Department of Psychology, Villanova University, Villanova, PA, USA

Amy Leonard Clay Department of Psychology, North Carolina State University, Raleigh, NC, USA

Staci M. Perlman Department of Human Development and Family Studies, University of Delaware, Newark, DE, USA

Timothy F. Piehler Department of Family Social Science, University of Minnesota, St. Paul, MN, USA

Molly Richard Center for Social Innovation, Needham Heights, MA, USA

Sara H. Shaw Department of Human Development and Family Studies, University of Delaware, Newark, DE, USA

Lauren A. Sparks Department of Psychology, Wayne State University, USA

Jennifer Tisdale The Salvation Army, Raleigh, NC, USA

Grace-Ann C. Whitney Connecticut Head Start Collaboration Office, Hartford, CT, USA

Chapter 1
Understanding and Meeting the Needs of Families Experiencing Homelessness: Introduction to the Brief

Mary E. Haskett

Introduction

Homelessness among US families has risen at a steady rate in recent decades and reached a peak during the recent recession. Families—most often single mothers with young children—are the fastest growing segment of the homeless population. Rates of homelessness are difficult to establish due to unreliable tracking and discrepancies in definitions across federal agencies. However, national experts estimate that approximately 2.5 million children were homeless in America in 2013 (Bassuk, DeCandia, Beach, & Berman, 2014); at this rate, Bassuk and colleagues propose that one in 30 US children experience a period of homelessness each year. Although there is wide variability in the experiences of families who suffer the loss of their home, and there are differences in adaptation of family members to those challenges, many parents and children who are homeless have faced adverse experiences that place them at risk for mental health and developmental concerns.

Author Note: This issue of *Advances in Child and Family Policy and Practice* is dedicated to Staci Perlman, MSW, Ph.D., our friend, mentor, and steadfast colleague in family homelessness. Dr. Perlman passed away after a brief illness in 2015. She was Assistant Professor of Human Development and Family Studies at the University of Delaware. Among her many professional roles, Dr. Perlman was a university professor who had the uncommon ability to work at micro and macro levels of influence simultaneously—on a single day, she could seamlessly transition from preparation of federal policy briefs to meetings with mothers and babies in shelters. Staci's unwavering dedication to young children and their parents struggling to provide the best for their children will continue in our work done in her honor and memory, including this Brief. *#yaybabies*.

M.E. Haskett (✉)
Department of Psychology, North Carolina State University, Box 7650,
Raleigh, NC 27695, USA
e-mail: mehasket@ncsu.edu

M.E. Haskett (ed.), *Child and Family Well-Being and Homelessness*,
SpringerBriefs in Psychology, DOI 10.1007/978-3-319-50886-3_1

Challenges Faced by Families Experiencing Homelessness

Prior to the period of homelessness, many children without homes have been exposed to violent incidents in their neighborhoods and families (Ponce, Lawless, & Rowe, 2014), they are less likely than housed children to have access to healthcare, and chronic health conditions are common (Cutuli et al., 2014). Many children without homes have been the subject of a child protection investigation, and rates of out-of-home placement are much higher than rates for the general population (David, Gelberg, & Suchman, 2012; Hoffman & Rosenheck, 2001). The cumulative risk experiences of children without homes are associated with high rates of mental health problems (Obradovic, 2010; Park, Fertig, & Allison, 2011). The federal McKinney-Vento Act provides homeless children with rights for educational stability, but many face disruptions in schooling and academic challenges (Masten et al., 2014; Obradovic et al., 2009).

Parents of children who experience homelessness tend to struggle with depression, substance abuse, and/or PTSD (Lee et al., 2010) and many have been involved in violent relationships (Browne, 1993; Ponce et al., 2014). A large proportion of mothers who are homelessness have faced traumatic events and depression occurs at a disproportionate rate (Bassuk & Beardslee, 2014). Parents who experience homelessness have difficulty providing sensitive caregiving for their children (e.g., Koblinsky, Morgan, & Anderson, 1997), report more frustration in the parenting role than housed mothers (Lee et al., 2010) and experience a high rate of involvement with child protective services and separations from their children (McChesney, 1995; Zlotnick, Kronstadt, & Klee, 1998).

After entering a shelter, the daily lives of parents and children can continue to be highly stressful. Although some housing programs provide excellent services to support families, shelter policies and the physical layout of the shelter are intended for safety rather than for support of positive parenting and healthy family interactions (e.g., Tischler, Rademeyer, & Vostanis, 2007). Housing facilities tend to be crowded and noisy, and they lack privacy and space for families to engage in their own routines and traditions (Friedman, 2000). Rarely are shelter policies sensitive to the needs of traumatized families. Low pay, limited job training, and job-related stress contribute to a high level of turnover among staff in housing programs (Olivet, McGraw, Grandin, & Bassuk, 2010). Finally, services provided to homeless families generally are not integrated or coordinated between housing agencies or across sectors (housing, education, job training, mental health) (Haber & Toro, 2004) so these clients might be more likely than stably housed clients to "fall through the cracks."

Purpose of This Issue

The purpose of this issue of *Advances in Child and Family Policy and Practice* is twofold. First, we aimed to increase awareness of the mental health, educational, and developmental challenges faced by children and their parents experiencing homelessness and to provide practice implications with a focus on assessment of functioning across domains and over time, individual differences in strengths and adjustment of parents and children experiencing homelessness, and innovative treatment and service delivery approaches. Second, we intended to advance a set of strong policy recommendations for assessment, intervention, research, and service delivery related to homeless children and their parents. These articles, authored by leading investigators and advocates in the field, highlight some of the most pressing challenges in addressing the needs of families who are experiencing homelessness.

Overview of the Contents

The vast majority of prior investigations of children experiencing homelessness have focused on the degree to which these children differ from housed children living in poverty. There has not been much attention to the individual differences among these children; for optimal prevention and intervention planning, such studies are essential. Janette Herbers and J.J. Cutuli and their colleagues lead the way in investigations of adaptation and resilience among children who have experienced the acute and potentially long-term stress of homelessness. In this issue, Herbers and her co-investigators share findings of a recent study designed to explore individual differences in mental health functioning *over time* among children experiencing an episode of homelessness. The authors consider the investigation to be a pilot study but the results and implications for practice are compelling nonetheless. Findings point to the importance of careful assessment of children and their parents across time to gain understanding of the unfolding nature of resilient functioning. As noted by the authors, this knowledge will aid in directing scarce services to children and families most at need, during the time they are likely to be most responsive to those services. As the number of families experiencing homelessness increases and funds for mental health services decrease in nearly every community across the county, studies such as this will become increasingly central in efforts to shape practices and policies for families experiencing homelessness.

The work of Kendal Holtrop and colleagues also addresses individual differences among families experiencing homelessness, with the goal of targeting parenting interventions to subgroups most likely to benefit. The research team's examinations of Early Risers for families transitioning out of homelessness represent some of the most carefully designed, programmatic studies in parenting interventions for families without homes. Holtrop and colleagues identified several factors that predicted positive responses to Early Risers. This is an intensive intervention, so identifying families most likely to benefit should allow agencies to direct limited resources to families at high risk, as defined by parental depression and more severe child behavior problems. "What works for which families?" is a critical question to address, but most extant research on parenting interventions for mothers and fathers experiencing homelessness is limited by small samples and lack of control groups (Haskett, Loehman, & Burkhart, 2014), thus, answering such complex questions about individual differences in response to treatment has not been possible. We hope Holtrop et al.'s investigation will serve as a model to move this research forward.

Identifying families with the most potential to benefit from particular services would require professionals to conduct at least a brief assessment of parent and child functioning. As demonstrated by Carmela DeCandia and her colleagues, such assessments are rarely conducted within housing programs. The authors, national leaders in research and advocacy in family homelessness, offer numerous recommendations to address this deep gap in services. This study points to the value of surveying front-line professionals in housing agencies to uncover strengths as well as deficiencies in services. Although the findings related to current assessment practices were generally discouraging, it is noteworthy that there were some programs (18%) considered "adequate" in assessment of child development and parent functioning. Our field should highlight those programs as models for housing providers around the country.

Staci Perlman and her colleagues also used a national survey of providers to understand another service challenge—accessing early childhood services for young children who are homeless. In addition to surveying providers, they also examined parent interview data collected to explore these issues from parents' points of view. By conducting analyses of two separate studies designed to address similar research questions, Perlman et al. provide a more comprehensive view of the issues than either study alone could have afforded. They identified variability in the degree to which housing providers were familiar with early childhood programs and frustration among parents regarding efforts to find high-quality, affordable, conveniently located programs for their children. This lack of accessibility could have devastating consequences for young children without homes because high-quality early childhood services could mitigate the developmental risks associated with homelessness. Perlman et al. argue persuasively for enhanced collaboration across service systems and better connections among parents, housing providers, and early childhood programs. They also suggest that a "point person" on the housing staff should be dedicated to assist families with the enrollment process.

Many of the recommendations put forth by Perlman and her coauthors are strategies implemented in Project CATCH, described in the article I coauthored with Tisdale and Leonard Clay. Our local community has had success in addressing some of the complex needs of children and parents experiencing homelessness (including accessing early childhood services) through cross-agency collaboration, sharing resources among housing agencies, and collectively advocating for family-serving agencies to reach homeless families. As recommended by DeCandia and colleagues, Project CATCH child case managers complete a fairly comprehensive screening and gather information from collateral sources to develop case management and treatment plans specific to children's needs. Of course, this is possible because there is a designated staff member (i.e., a point person) to focus on the children's functioning and individual needs. Although Project CATCH was developed to meet many of the challenges addressed by the authors of papers in this issue, there remain challenges and gaps in services in our community. Critical to closing some of the most significant gaps will be public policies that encourage and *fund* housing providers to support families whose needs for stability extend beyond housing. Preston Britner and Anne Farrell summarize practice and policy recommendations derived from the results of this set of papers. We are optimistic that those recommendations will resonate with practitioners and researchers, and—most importantly—that policy makers will heed their pointed recommendations.

References

Bassuk, E. L., & Beardslee, W. R. (2014). Depression in homeless mothers: Addressing an unrecognized public health issue. *American Journal of Orthopsychiatry, 84*, 73–81. doi:10.1037/h0098949.

Bassuk, E. L., DeCandia, C. J., Beach, C., & Berman, F. (2014). *America's youngest outcasts: A report card on child homelessness*. Waltham, MA: The National Center on Family Homelessness at AIR.

Browne, A. (1993). Family violence and homelessness: The relevance of trauma histories in the lives of homeless women. *American Journal of Orthopsychiatry, 63*, 370–383. doi:10.1037/h0079444.

Cutuli, J. J., Herbers, J. E., Lafavor, T. L., Ahumada, S. M., Masten, A. S., & Oberg, C. N. (2014). Asthma and adaptive functioning among homeless kindergarten-aged children in emergency housing. *Journal of Health Care for the Poor and Underserved, 25*, 717–730. doi:10.1353/hpu.2014.0099.

David, D. H., Gelberg, L., & Suchman, N. E. (2012). Implications of homelessness for parenting young children: A preliminary review from a developmental attachment perspective. *Infant Mental Health Journal, 33*, 1–9. doi:10.1002/imhj.20333.

Friedman, D. H. (2000). *Parenting in public*. New York, NY: Columbia University Press.

Haber, M. G., & Toro, P. A. (2004). Homelessness among families, children, and adolescents: An ecological-developmental perspective. *Clinical Child and Family Psychology Review, 7*, 123–164. doi:10.1023/B:CCFP.0000045124.09503.fl.

Haskett, M. E., Loehman, J., & Burkhart, K. (2014). Parenting interventions in shelter settings: A qualitative systematic review of the literature. *Child & Family Social Work, 21*, 272–282.

Hoffman, D., & Rosenheck, R. (2001). Homeless mothers with severe mental illness and their children: Predictors of family reunification. *Psychiatric Rehabilitation Journal, 25*, 163–169. doi:10.1037/h0095029.

Koblinsky, S. A., Morgan, K. M., & Anderson, E. A. (1997). African-American homeless and low-income housed mothers: Comparison of parenting practices. *American Journal of Orthopsychiatry, 67*, 37–47. doi:10.1037/h0080209.

Lee, S. S., August, G. J., Gewirtz, A. H., Klimes-Dougan, B., Bloomquist, M. L., & Realmuto, G. (2010). Identifying unmet mental health needs of children of formerly homeless mothers living in a supportive housing community sector of care. *Journal of Abnormal Child Psychology, 38*, 421–432. doi:10.1007/s10802-009-9378-1.

Masten, A. S., Cutuli, J. J., Herbers, J. E., Hinz, E., Obradovic, J., & Wenzel, A. J. (2014). Academic risk and resilience in the context of homelessness. *Child Development Perspectives*, *8*, 201–206. doi:10.1111/cdep.12088.

McChesney, K. Y. (1995). A review of the empirical literature on contemporary urban homeless families. *Social Service Review*, *69*, 429–460.

Obradovic, J. (2010). Effortful control and adaptive functioning of homeless children: Variable-focused and person-focused analyses. *Journal of Applied Developmental Psychology*, *31*, 109–117. doi:10.1016/j.appdev.2009.09.004.

Obradovic, J., Long, J. D., Cutuli, J. J., Chan, A., Hinz, E., & Heisted, D. (2009). Academic achievement of homeless and highly mobile children in an urban school district: Longitudinal evidence of risk, growth and resilience. *Development and Psychopathology*, *21*, 493–518. doi:10.1017/S0954579409000273.

Olivet, J., McGraw, S., Grandin, M., & Bassuk, E. (2010). Staffing challenges and strategies for organizations serving individuals who have experienced chronic homelessness. *Journal of Behavioral Health Services & Research*, *37*, 226–238. doi:10.1007/s1414-009-9201-3.

Park, J., Fertig, A., & Allison, P. (2011). Physical and mental health, cognitive development, and health care use by housing status of low-income young children in 20 American cities: A prospective cohort study. *American Journal of Public Health*, *101*, S255–S261. doi:10.1080/01488376.2015.1018660.

Ponce, A. N., Lawless, M. S., & Rowe, M. (2014). Homelessness, behavioral health disorders and intimate partner violence: barriers to services for women. *Community Mental Health Journal*, *50*, 831–840. doi:10.1007/s10597-014-9712-0.

Tischler, V., Rademeyer, A., & Vostanis, P. (2007). Mothers experiencing homelessness: Mental health, support, and social care needs. *Health & Social Care in the Community*, *15*, 246–253. doi:10.1111/j.1365-2524.2206.00678.x.

Zlotnick, C., Kronstadt, D., & Klee, L. (1998). Foster care children and family homelessness. *American Journal of Public Health*, *88*, 1368–1370. doi:10.2105/AJPH.88.1.1368.

Chapter 2
Mental Health and Adaptation of Children Experiencing Family Homelessness

Janette E. Herbers, J.J. Cutuli, Lyuboslava Kolarova, Amanda Albu, and Lauren A. Sparks

Introduction

Family homelessness is a context of risk for children (Buckner, 2008; Samuels, Shinn, & Buckner, 2010). While the challenges and needs of many children experiencing family homelessness are substantial, so too are their strengths. These strengths allow a good number of children to demonstrate resilience despite homelessness (Bassuk, Richard, & Tsertsvadze, 2015; Cutuli & Herbers, 2014; Cutuli et al., 2013; Haskett, Armstrong, & Tisdale, 2015; Masten et al., 2014; Obradovic, 2010). If we can better understand how children and families successfully adapt to episodes of homelessness, we can apply those lessons to develop better policies, practices, and social service systems to support those who struggle (Cutuli & Herbers, 2014). To gain and then apply this knowledge, researchers as well as providers need ways to differentiate between the children and families who already possess the strengths necessary to adapt versus those who need more support from interventions. This can lead to more successful, cost-effective, and efficient approaches to social services (Bassuk, Volk, & Olivet, 2010; Cutuli & Herbers, 2014; Haskett et al., 2015; Huntington, Buckner, & Bassuk, 2008). In this report, we present findings from a pilot study designed to assess short-term processes of adaptation in school-age children and their parents during a stay in

J.E. Herbers, Ph.D. (✉) • L. Kolarova
Department of Psychology, Villanova University, Villanova, PA, USA
e-mail: Janette.Herbers@villanova.edu

J.J. Cutuli
Department of Psychology, Rutgers University—Camden, Camden, NJ, USA

A. Albu
Office of Institutional Research and Assessment, Temple University, USA

L.A. Sparks
Department of Psychology, Wayne State University, USA

M.E. Haskett (ed.), *Child and Family Well-Being and Homelessness*,
SpringerBriefs in Psychology, DOI 10.1007/978-3-319-50886-3_2

emergency housing, with an emphasis on assessment of child mental health and factors that may predict mental health problems.

Resilience science is guided by broader developmental theory, and has been the topic of rigorous research for the past 50 years (see Cutuli, Herbers, Masten, & Reed, in press; Masten & Cicchetti, in press). Consistently throughout the decades of this science, individuals vary in their responses to adversity; some suffer significant difficulties while others weather the threats, demonstrating healthy functioning either throughout or within a relatively brief period of time following adverse experiences (Masten, 2001; Masten et al., 2014; Rutter, 2013). Families who seek emergency housing often do so following a traumatic or highly stressful event, such as an incident of domestic or community violence, eviction from their previous home, or a falling out with friends or relatives with whom they were residing (Anooshian, 2005; Cowan, 2014; Perlman, Cowan, Gewirtz, Haskett, & Stokes, 2012). In addition, it is common for these children and parents to have multiple stressful events in their histories, particularly within the past year (Cutuli & Herbers, 2014; Masten, Miliotis, Graham-Bermann, Ramirez, & Neemann, 1993). Thus the move to emergency housing for many represents an acute stressor in the context of a complex history of past adversities and ongoing poverty-related stress.

Resilience science describes several different patterns of adaptation based on how individuals function before, during, and after adversity (see Cutuli et al., in press; Southwick, Bonanno, Masten, Panter-Brick, & Yehuda, 2014). Applied to the adversities of family homelessness, those who show a stress-resistant pattern have good functioning before, during, and after entering emergency housing. These individuals and families should be fairly easy to identify with appropriate assessment tools. A second, distinct pattern of resilience involves a period of disrupted or suboptimal functioning followed by a rebound to typical levels in a reasonable amount of time. Sometimes this pattern is referred to as "bouncing back" and is largely the product of various protective factors like close, positive relationships, better self-regulation and cognitive functioning, and other supports within the individual, family, or community (Cutuli et al., in press; Luthar, Crossman, & Small, 2015; Masten & Cicchetti, in press). Recognizing this second pattern of resilience in its early stages poses a greater challenge. Initially, these children and families will likely resemble those who will continue to have problems and maintain maladaptive trajectories. However, there are clear implications for social policy and practice; if we can differentiate families who will bounce back using the protective factors already in their lives, it will allow providers to focus on others who are unlikely to show resilience without intervention. Limited resources for more intensive services then could be allocated to the families who need them most. Also and at least as important, for families in the process of successful adaptation, the best approach of service systems may be to minimize unnecessary interference, empowering parents and maintaining a sense of normalcy for children. Well-intentioned programs might inadvertently undermine important protective factors in families' lives, like parental self-efficacy, family routines, and a swift departure from institutional living, thereby interfering with natural processes of resilience (Perlman et al., 2012).

To understand how positive adaptation occurs in the context of homelessness, it is necessary to assess functioning over time. Though longitudinal studies of well-being in homeless children are few, some have demonstrated patterns of recovery in academic achievement following episodes of homelessness (Cutuli et al., 2013; Rafferty, Shinn, & Weitzman, 2004). With regard to mental health, many studies have documented high rates of problems among children experiencing family homelessness (Bassuk et al., 2015; Cowan, 2014; Samuels et al., 2010). Shinn et al. (2008) followed up with two groups of families—one group had been homeless about 4 or 5 years prior and the other poor-but-housed at the time. They found inconsistent evidence that children who had been homeless had more mental health symptoms than the comparison group. No differences were found among adolescents; formerly homeless children between the ages of 7 and 10 years had more symptoms as a function of other stressors they had experienced, and children who were between the ages of 4–6 years had more mental health problems. Little else is known about how these problems may change over time both during and following homeless episodes. It is possible that assessing children's mental health near the time of shelter entry, an acute crisis for the family, could yield unreliable and misleading information. Children in the early phases of a "bouncing back" trajectory could appear maladaptive for a time, but that profile would not represent their eventual resilient functioning. Whether such improvements may be evident during the course of a stay in emergency housing is unknown.

Another relevant aspect of assessing child mental health is measurement. As in many other service settings, it is likely that most information gathered by providers in emergency housing is solicited from the parents, including information about child well-being or problems (Kisiel, Conradi, Fehrenbach, Torgersen, & Briggs, 2014). However, like their children, parents in this context are in the midst of acute adversity and may have difficulty providing accurate accounts of their children's symptoms. Following traumatic events, there tend to be substantial discrepancies between parents' and children's reports of child symptoms, particularly for older children and particularly regarding internalizing problems. Parents often underestimate children's symptoms of traumatic stress (Shemesh et al., 2005; Stover, Hahn, Berkowitz, & Im, 2010). Furthermore, parents' reports of child symptoms can be associated more strongly with parents' own distress than with children's self-reported symptoms (Kassam-Adams, Garcia-Espana, Miller, & Winston, 2006). Since families in emergency housing often have histories of trauma in addition to stressors associated with homelessness, parents coping with their own distress in emergency housing may confound their subjective feelings with their perceptions of their children's functioning. Accurate assessment might require seeking information from other sources, including self-report from children old enough to provide it.

Besides or in addition to repeated assessments of mental health, how else might practitioners and service providers identify the children most likely to bounce back? Resilience science points to a robust set of protective factors that tend to predict healthy child functioning in the face of a broad range of risky and adverse circumstances. In particular, children at risk benefit from two central adaptive systems: good cognitive functioning in the forms of both general intelligence

(IQ) and executive functioning (EF), and positive relationships with parents or other caregivers (Luthar et al., 2015; Masten, 2001, 2014). IQ and EF abilities are aspects of cognitive functioning that are related but distinct (Garon, Bryson, & Smith, 2008; Masten et al., 2012). EF refers to a set of metacognitive abilities involved in cognitive control of attention, thoughts, and behaviors in the service of accomplishing goals (Best & Miller, 2010; Diamond & Lee, 2011). Difficulties with EF predict mental health problems in children and youth, with stronger associations with externalizing problems such as aggression and hyperactivity than with internalizing problems such as anxiety and depression (Hughes & Ensor, 2011; Riggs, Jahromi, Razza, Dillworth-Bart, & Mueller, 2006; Wagner, Alloy, & Abramson, 2015). Exposure to trauma has been associated with EF difficulties as well (DePrince, Weinzierl, & Combs, 2009).

EF and other aspects of self-regulation and cognitive functioning develop in the context of parent–child relationships (Bernier, Carlson, & Whipple, 2010; Calkins & Hill, 2007; Herbers, Cutuli, Supkoff, Narayan, & Masten, 2014). Parenting that involves warmth, responsiveness, and appropriate discipline is associated with child mental health, and positive parent–child relationships are considered the most robust protective factor in a variety of adverse circumstances (Luthar & Brown, 2007; Luthar et al., 2015; Masten, 2014). Both cognitive functioning and positive parenting have demonstrated associations with children's well-being within samples of children experiencing homelessness (Buckner, Mezzacappa, & Beardslee, 2003, 2009; Herbers et al., 2014; Herbers et al., 2011; Masten et al., 2012; Obradovic, 2010; Piehler et al., 2014) and are recommended targets for interventions aiming to improve these families' outcomes (Bassuk, DeCandia, Beach, & Berman, 2014).

To further understand how children adapt in the context of family emergency housing, and how aspects of measurement might obscure positive adaptation, we defined three specific goals for this study. First, we aimed to describe children's mental health symptoms measured at two time points, 1 month apart during their stay in emergency housing. With well-validated measures of parent distress and child traumatic stress, internalizing problems, and externalizing problems, we expected to find improvements across the 1-month interval based on both child report and parent report. For our second goal, we were interested in comparing children's self-reported and parent-reported traumatic stress symptoms in the context of parent distress, with the expectation that parents would conflate their own distress with their perceptions of children's traumatic stress, leading to inaccurate reports particularly by the most distressed parents. Finally, we sought to predict mental health outcomes after one month from specific factors that vary across individuals and families: child cognitive functioning including general intelligence and executive functioning, and warmth expressed by parents regarding their children.

Method

Participants and Procedures

Children between the ages of 8–11 years and their parents (i.e., primary caregivers) were recruited for participation while staying in two emergency shelters in West Philadelphia. In order to be eligible, children and caregivers had to be fluent in English, children could not have previously identified disabilities that would interfere with performance on study tasks, and families had to have been in residence at the shelter for at least three nights to give them time to acclimate. Only one child per family could participate; in families with two or more eligible children, the youngest eligible child was selected. One parent (the primary caregiver) from each family participated. All recruitment and data collection sessions occurred onsite at the shelters in accordance with protocols established through collaboration with the housing providers and staff, and with IRB approval through Villanova University and Rutgers University-Camden. Parents provided written consent and children gave written assent.

Participation involved two 60 min sessions, an initial (T1) and one-month follow-up (T2), as well as three brief weekly check-ins spaced between T1 and T2. Data from the check-ins involved information regarding physical health that was part of a larger study not relevant to this report. For the T1 and T2 sessions, parents completed a structured interview with one researcher while children completed cognitive assessments and questionnaires with another researcher in a separate room. All measures were administered by interview with researchers recording responses in order to be sensitive to differences in literacy. Parents received $20 in gift cards and children received toys as honoraria at the completion of each session.

A total of 19 children completed a T1 session with their parents, representing 70.4% of eligible families during the study period. Fourteen (73.7%) completed the T2 session one month following their T1. Of the initial 19, ten children were female and nine male. On average, children were 9 years, 5 months old (SD = 13 months) and parents were 35 years, 8 months old (SD = 8 years, 3 months). All parents were female, and the majority were biological parents of the target children. According to parent report, 14 children were identified as African-American and the remaining children were identified as having multiracial or "other" ethnic backgrounds. Sixty-three percent of parents reported that they had previously stayed with relatives or friends, and the most common reasons endorsed for seeking shelter were being unable to afford rent (47.4%), evicted from housing (31.6%), laid off from a job (36.8%), or relationship problems (36.8%). Most parents indicated government funds as their main source of income.

Measures

Traumatic Stress

Children's symptoms of traumatic stress were measured at T1 and T2 both by self-report and parent report using the UCLA PTSD Reaction Index for DSM-IV (Pynoos, Rodriguez, Steinberg, Stuber, & Frederick, 1998). Children responded to 22 items assessing the frequency of their trauma-related symptoms using a five-point Likert scale ranging from 0 = "none in the past month" to 4 = "most days in the past month." Parents responded to 21 items regarding their children's trauma-related symptoms with the same scale. Scores from the items were summed separately to create overall severity scores, one based on child report and one from parent report. The measures also were scored according to the algorithm for determining whether the configuration and severity of symptoms met criteria for a diagnosis of post-traumatic stress disorder (PTSD) based on DSM-IV. In other words, children were identified as likely meeting criteria for PTSD if they had at least one re-experiencing symptom, three avoidance symptoms, and two increased arousal symptoms endorsed with severity of 3 or 4.

Internalizing Problems

Children's internalizing problems were assessed at both T1 and T2 via self-report and parent report. Symptoms of depression were measured with the Children's Depression Inventory, Second Edition (CDI-2: Kovacs, 2011), a self-report measure with 28 items assessing depression symptoms in youth ages 7–17 years. On each item, children selected one from a list of three statements that best described their feelings. The sets of statements were assigned point values based on severity, and the sums of all items were converted to T-scores adjusted for age and gender. T-scores at or above 65 are considered clinically significant (Kovacs, 2003), and dummy codes were created to indicate scores above this threshold.

Parents completed the parent-report form of the Strengths and Difficulties Questionnaire (SDQ: Goodman, 1997). The SDQ consists of 25 items comprising five items for each of the following subscales: emotional symptoms, conduct problems, hyperactivity/inattention, peer relationship problems, and prosocial behavior. The emotional symptoms subscale includes items representing symptoms of depression ("often unhappy, depressed, or tearful") and anxiety ("many worries or often seems worried"), and thus was selected as a parent report of general internalizing problems. Each item has a three-point response set with 0 = "not true," 1 = "somewhat true," and 2 = "certainly true." Item scores were summed to create the emotional symptoms score. Emotional symptoms scores above 5 were coded to represent "high difficulties" with significant clinical risk (Bourdon, Goodman, Rae, Simpson, & Koretz, 2005).

Externalizing Problems

The conduct problems and prosocial (reversed) subscales of the SDQ were utilized to measure children's externalizing problems via parent report. Items from each individual subscale were summed separately then scores were combined as an average of the conduct problems and reverse-scored prosocial scales ($\alpha = .79$ at T1, $\alpha = .68$ at T2). A dummy code for "high difficulties" was created based on established cut-points (above 3 for conduct problems and below 4 for prosocial), such that a child meeting the cutoff for either or both subscales was coded "1."

Executive Functioning (EF)

At both T1 and T2, children used a touchscreen tablet to complete the computerized version of the *Dimensional Change Card Sort* (DCCS: Zelazo, 2006) as a measure of executive functioning. The DCCS requires children to follow and switch rules when matching target images to stimuli according to different categories (Zelazo, 2006). The task includes 40 trials that alternate between sorting by shape and by color. Computer software records accuracy and response time. The task was administered using E-Prime software (Schneider, Eschman, & Zuccolotto, 2012) and also is part of the NIH Toolbox Cognition Battery (National-Institute-of-Health, 2011; Zelazo, Anderson, & Richler, 2011). Scores are computed based on accuracy to post-switch trials with reaction time incorporated when accuracy is above 73.3% (NIH, 2011). We include only the T1 assessment as longitudinal patterns of responses suggest complex measurement characteristics beyond the scope of the current paper.

Intellectual Functioning (IQ)

Children's intellectual functioning was assessed at T1 and T2, using subscales from two comparable measures that were counterbalanced such that about half the children completed each measure at each time point. Both measures were Wechsler scales—the Wechsler Intelligence Scale for Children, Fourth Edition (WISC-IV: Wechsler, 2003), and the Wechsler Abbreviated Scales of Intelligence, Second Edition (WASI-II: Wechsler & Hsiao-pin, 2011). The Vocabulary and Matrix Reasoning subscales were used to estimate verbal and performance IQ, respectively. Raw scores were converted to scale scores ($M = 10$, SD = 3). Scores on Vocabulary and Matrix Reasoning were moderately correlated ($r = .55$ at T1, $r = .54$ at T2) and were averaged at each time point to create estimates of general IQ.

Parenting Warmth

As a measure of parenting warmth, parents completed the Five Minute Speech Sample (FMSS: Magana et al., 1986) at T1 and T2. The FMSS is a brief measure of expressed emotion that has been used with a wide variety of populations, including parents of children experiencing homelessness, and has demonstrated validity for predicting parenting behaviors and children's adjustment difficulties (Narayan, Herbers, Plowman, Gewirtz, & Masten, 2012; Sher-Censor, 2015). Parents were asked to speak for five minutes, describing what kind of person their child is and how they get along. A list of standardized prompts were used to assist parents who had difficulty speaking spontaneously for the full duration. Audio-recordings were later coded for expressed warmth and negativity based on content of statements and affective tone (Caspi et al., 2004). Both the warmth and negativity codes were rated on scales from 0–5 by two independent raters who were blind to other aspects of the participants and data, including time point. Inter-rater reliability was very good with ICCs = .87 for warmth and .75 for negativity. Scores from the two coders were averaged, then the warmth scores and reversed negativity scores were averaged as a composite ($\alpha = .87$ at T1; $\alpha = .66$ at T2).

Parent Distress

Parents reported their own levels of distress at both T1 and T2 using a brief version of the Hopkins Symptom Checklist (SCL-25; Derogatis, Lipman, Rickels, Uhlenhuth, & Covi, 1974), which includes 13 items related to symptoms of depression, 2 items reflecting somatization, and 10 items related to anxiety. Parents indicated the degree to which they had experienced each symptom in the past week, on a scale from 1 to 4 with 1 = "not at all" and 4 = "extremely." Items include "feeling everything is an effort," "feeling no interest in things," and "feeling tense or keyed up." Scores for all items were averaged as a continuous measure of current distress. Dummy codes were assigned to indicate clinically elevated scores based on the recommended clinical cutoff of 1.75 (Sandanger et al., 1998).

Missing Data

As mentioned previously, 14 out of 19 families completed the T2 session, yielding 26.3% missing data across T2 measures. There were no indications that missing data patterns departed from missing-at-random assumptions, and we employed multiple imputations using the recommended multichain Monte Carlo algorithm with fully conditional specification (Schafer & Graham, 2002) in IBM SPSS Statistics 22. Data were imputed 20 times creating 20 different datasets, with results of analyses on the 20 datasets combined according to Rubin's Rules (Rubin, 1987). Imputed data are presented in all tables and figures.

Results

Rates and Changes in Mental Health Problems

The first goal of the study was to examine rates of children's and parents' mental health symptoms at the initial and one-month follow-up time points. Using clinical cutoff points across all the child mental health measures, we determined that at T1, 31.6% of children had no clinically elevated scores. This number increased to 42.1% at T2, and the difference in counts over time was statistically significant ($\chi^2 = 4.97$, $p = .026$).

For each individual measure, rates and possible changes were considered based on continuous mean scores as well as categorical scoring indicating clinical cutoff points or diagnostic coding (see Fig. 2.1). Means, standard deviations, and rates based on categorical scoring are listed in Table 2.1. We tested for mean differences using paired samples t-tests and for count changes using chi-squares and Fisher's exact test for significance within a small sample.

At T1, the average score on the UCLA PTSD Reaction Index was 30.3 (SD = 16.4) based on child report and 15.2 (SD = 10.2) based on parent report. Both scores were somewhat lower at T2, though the mean differences across the month were not statistically significant based on paired samples T-tests for either measure ($t = 1.29$, $p = .199$ and $t = 1.49$, $p = .136$, respectively). According to child report on the measure, 31.6% met the measure's criteria for likely PTSD diagnosis at T1

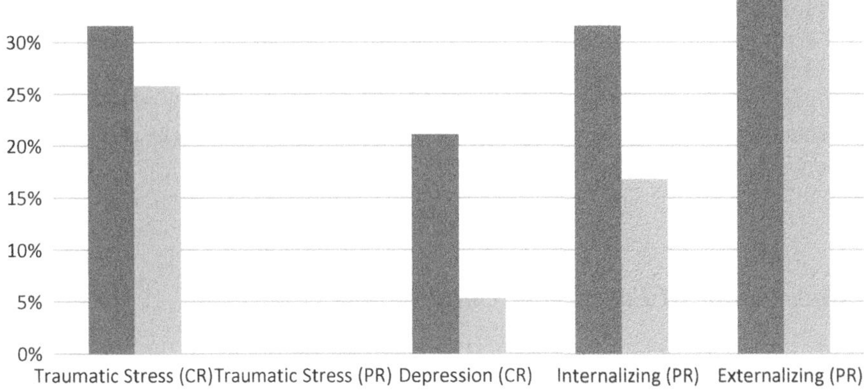

Fig. 2.1 Rates of children's mental health problems at T1 and T2. *CR* = child self-report, *PR* = parent report

Table 2.1 Means, standard deviations, and percentages above clinical cutoffs for measures of child mental health and parent distress

	Time 1		Time 2	
	M (SD)	% clinical	*M* (SD)	% clinical
Traumatic stress-CR	30.3 (16.4)	31.6	26.1 (11.9)	25.8
Traumatic stress-PR	15.2 (10.2)	0.0	12.5 (6.14)	0.0
Depression-CR	56.4 (12.1)	21.1	53.5 (8.62)	5.3
Internalizing-PR	2.47 (2.74)	31.6	1.59 (1.72)	16.8
Externalizing-PR	1.95 (2.21)	42.1	1.94 (1.35)	46.8
Parent distress-PR	1.95 (0.72)	52.6	1.82 (0.66)	41.0

Notes: *CR* child self-report, *PR* parent report

and 25.8% met those criteria at T2. This difference was not statistically significant ($\chi^2 = 1.45$, $p = .505$). At both T1 and T2, none of the parent reports met the measure's criteria for likely PTSD diagnosis.

Scores based on child report of depression symptoms on the CDI-2 had means significantly above the population average at both T1 ($M = 56.4$, SD = 12.1; $t = 2.32$, $p = .016$) and T2 ($M = 53.5$, SD = 8.62; $t = 1.77$, $p = .047$). The mean difference across time points was not significant ($t = 1.39$, $p = .163$). At T1, 21.1% had T-scores above 65 vs. 5.3% at T2, though the pattern was not statistically significant ($\chi^2 = 3.96$, $p = .211$).

According to parent report, average scores for children's internalizing and externalizing problems fell below the threshold for "high difficulties" at both time points (see Table 2.1). Scores on parent-reported internalizing problems showed a statistical trend with lower scores at T2 than at T1 ($t = 1.86$, $p = .063$). Considering counts, 31.6% of internalizing scores fell above the high difficulties threshold at T1 compared to 16.8% at T2, a significant difference ($\chi^2 = 7.72$, $p = .005$). There was no significant mean difference in parent-reported externalizing problems across the time points ($t = 0.76$, $p = .979$). Counts of children meeting the high difficulties threshold for externalizing problems increased from 42.1% at T1 to 46.8% at T2, a significant difference ($\chi^2 = 11.9$, $p < .001$).

Finally, parent reports of their own distress on the SCL-25 had average scores above the clinical cutoff both at T1 ($M = 1.95$, SD = 0.72) and T2 ($M = 1.82$, SD = 0.66) with no significant mean difference from T1 to T2 ($t = .797$, $p = .426$). Based on counts, 52.6% were above the threshold at T1 and 41.0% were above at T2, which is a statistically significant difference ($\chi^2 = 6.07$, $p = .038$).

Concordance of Parent and Child Report

For our second goal, we examined the associations between parent and child reports of children's mental health problems and tested the hypothesis that parents' reports of child problems would be related to parent distress. Correlations among continuous scores for the measures are presented in Table 2.2. The association between

Table 2.2 Bivariate correlations of measures of child mental health and parent distress at T1 and T2

	1	2	3	4	5	6	7	8	9
1. T1 Traumatic stress (CR)	–								
2. T2 Traumatic stress (CR)	.538*	–							
3. T1 Traumatic stress (PR)	.378	.164	–						
4. T2 Traumatic stress (PR)	.236	.029	.668**	–					
5. T1 Depression (CR)	.540*	.447	.364	.196	–				
6. T2 Depression (CR)	.489*	.614**	.300	.141	.675**	–			
7. T1 Internalizing (PR)	.093	.188	.792**	.592*	.289	.239	–		
8. T2 Internalizing (PR)	.354	.310	.611*	.586**	.199	.338	.687**	–	
9. T1 Externalizing (PR)	.113	−.318	.186	.004	−.387	−.169	−.078	−.067	–
10. T2 Externalizing (PR)	.195	−.320	.087	.074	−.338	−.251	−.140	.066	.679**

Notes: *CR* child self-report, *PR* parent report
*$p < .05$; **$p < .01$

child report of depression symptoms and parent report of child internalizing problems was low-to-moderate but not significant at T1 ($r = .289$, $p = .234$) and T2 ($r = .338$, $p = .164$). At T1, parent self-reported distress was significantly correlated with parent report of children's internalizing problems ($r = .601$, $p = .005$) but not with parent report of children's externalizing problems ($r = .264$, $p = .280$) or children's self-reported depression symptoms ($r = .247$, $p = .327$). These patterns were generally consistent within T2 measures as well (see Table 2.2).

At T1, the correlation between children's self-reported traumatic stress symptoms and parent-reported traumatic stress symptoms was moderate but not significant ($r = .378$, $p = .112$). At T2, the correlation between these two measures was nonsignificant with an effect size of nearly zero ($r = .029$, $p = .909$). Mean differences in continuous traumatic stress scores between self-report and parent report were significant both at T1 ($t = 4.20$, $p < .001$) and T2 ($t = 4.41$, $p < .001$). Parents, on average, reported lower levels of traumatic stress symptoms for their children. Parent self-reported distress was significantly correlated with parent-reported child traumatic stress symptoms ($r = .658$, $p = .007$) but not child-reported traumatic stress ($r = .135$, $p = .590$).

To test more rigorously whether parent-reported traumatic stress reflected parent distress, we regressed parent-reported traumatic stress symptoms (for the child) on child self-reported traumatic stress symptoms in one step of a linear regression, then added parent self-reported distress in the second step. We did this twice, once for T1 and once for T2 scores. We considered the R-square change in each step. In the first step of the T1 model, child self-reported traumatic stress accounted for 14.3% of the variance in parent-reported traumatic stress and was not a significant predictor ($B = .235$, SE*[B]* $= .139$, $p = .111$). When added, parent distress accounted for an additional 28.0% of the variance and emerged as a significant predictor ($B = 7.46$, SE*[B]* $= 2.68$, $p = .013$). In the T2 model, child self-reported traumatic stress accounted for 0.1% of the variance in child traumatic stress reported by the parent in the first step. Parent distress accounted for an additional 43.3% of the variance and emerged as significant in the second step ($B = 6.17$, SE*[B]* $= 2.09$, $p = .004$).

Finally, to examine whether parents experiencing less distress were more accurate in reporting their children's symptoms of traumatic stress, we examined the correlation between parent-reported traumatic stress symptoms and children's self-reported traumatic stress symptoms separately for parents below and above the clinical cutoff on the SCL-25 at each time point. At T1, for parents who scored in the clinical range, the correlation was $r = .147$, $p = .696$. For parents who scored below the clinical range, the correlation was $r = .693$, $p = .039$. The difference between these two correlations is moderate in effect size but not statistically significant ($z = 1.27$, $p = .102$). At T2, the correlation between parent and child report for parents who scored in the clinical range was $r = -.357$, $p = .442$. For parents who scored below, the correlation was $r = -.047$, $p = .896$. The difference in magnitude of correlations was not significant ($z = 0.57$, $p = .284$).

Predictors of Mental Health

To test whether executive functioning, intellectual functioning, and positive parenting measured at T1 would predict child mental health a month later at T2, we ran a series of multiple linear regressions with T2 measures of traumatic stress symptoms (child self-report), depression (child self-report), and externalizing problems (parent report) as outcomes. We did not include parent-reported child traumatic stress symptoms or child internalizing problems as outcomes based our expectation from the literature that these reports would be less accurate than their reports of externalizing problems. Age and gender were included as control variables.

In the model predicting child self-reported traumatic stress symptoms, the only significant predictor was EF ($B = 4.34$, SE$[B] = 1.92$, $p = .024$), such that higher scores predicted higher levels of traumatic stress symptoms. Overall, the model explained 39.8% of the variance in traumatic stress symptoms. The same pattern emerged in the model predicting child self-reported depression symptoms, with EF as the only significant predictor ($B = 2.83$, SE$[B] = 1.37$, $p = .038$). This model explained 43.7% of the variance in depression symptoms.

In the model predicting parent-reported externalizing problems, age emerged as statistically significant ($B = -.754$, SE$[B] = .266$, $p = .005$) as did parenting warmth ($B = -.538$, SE$[B] = .255$, $p = .035$), with younger children showing more problems and parenting warmth associated with fewer problems. There was a trend indicating that children with higher EF scores had fewer externalizing problems ($B = -.296$, SE$[B] = .174$, $p = .089$).

Discussion

Generally speaking, 8- to 11-year-olds in emergency family housing were at risk for mental health problems, though a noteworthy percentage were functioning well. The number of children demonstrating resilience with respect to mental health increased significantly over the course of 1 month. Fewer parents reported clinical levels of distress after 1 month as well, suggesting that some are adapting well despite homelessness. These children and parents likely represent two patterns of resilient functioning, those who maintain good functioning throughout adverse experiences and those who show improvements following a brief period of difficulty.

Still, homelessness represents a context of noteworthy risk. Elevated rates of mental health problems found in this study are consistent with the broader literature on families experiencing homelessness (Bassuk et al., 2014, 2015; Cowan, 2014). Nearly half of children in the sample scored within the high difficulties range based on parent report of externalizing problems, like defiance and aggression. Average scores for depression symptoms based on self-report fell above population means, and nearly one-third of children met criteria for a likely PTSD diagnosis based on children's own accounts of their thoughts and feelings.

Parent and Child Perceptions of Internalizing Symptoms

As we expected, parents' reports of their own distress appear linked to their perceptions of their children's functioning, at least for internalizing symptoms and traumatic stress. Parents generally underreported symptoms for their children when their own distress was high. Not only were parent-reported scores of child traumatic stress significantly lower than those reported by the children, but strikingly, none of the parent-reported scores met criteria for PTSD. Parent distress predicted parent-reported child traumatic stress symptoms better than child self-reported traumatic stress. These findings suggest that many parents are failing to recognize their children's substantial traumatic stress symptoms, partly due to their own subjective experiences.

An interesting caveat has to do with our finding that many parents' own symptoms seem to improve over the course of a month, meaning that their subjective distress and internalizing symptoms decrease. While parents reported decreased internalizing symptoms for their children after one month, there was no significant change in children's self-reported depression or traumatic stress symptoms. It seems unlikely that parents become more accurate reporters of child internalizing and traumatic stress symptoms as their own symptoms improve. As an alternative, perhaps children are less likely to recognize and/or report improvements in their own functioning over time. Another possibility is that parents could be reporting fewer problems at follow-up, regardless of whom they are describing. This, too, is unlikely because parents reported about the same level of child externalizing symptoms at the first assessment and one month later. Rather, it may be that parents have particular difficulty recognizing child symptoms of certain types, namely internalizing and traumatic stress symptoms.

For parents to be less accurate in their reports of child internalizing problems and traumatic stress is not unique to families experiencing homelessness. Reports from other populations describe the same or a similar phenomenon (Kassam-Adams et al., 2006; Meiser-Stedman, Smith, Glucksman, Yule, & Dalgleish, 2007; Shemesh et al., 2005; Stover et al., 2010). Internalizing symptoms generally involve mood problems, be they related to anxiety or depression, which either lack external displays or have displays that may be misinterpreted as externalizing symptoms without underlying dysregulation of mood. For those focused on family homelessness, this phenomenon has implications relevant to practice and policy decision-making. When responding to calls for routine assessments of trauma and traumatic stress among children experiencing homelessness, and for intervention strategies that target sequelae of trauma (Bassuk et al., 2014), it is important to include information from sources other than parents. It is especially important to ask children about their own experiences when developmentally appropriate (Kisiel et al., 2014). Doing so will open a window into the child's internal state of emotions that, according to our findings, seem more difficult for parents to recognize.

Protective Factors

Both executive functioning and parents' expressed warmth towards their children predicted fewer externalizing behavior problems at T2, as expected. Executive functions can aid in cognitive control of thoughts, emotions, and behaviors, with well-established implications for symptoms of psychopathology (Snyder, Miyake, & Hankin, 2015). Poor EF particularly has been linked with externalizing problems, especially ones related to aggression and impulsivity (see Hughes & Ensor, 2011; Ogilvie, Stewart, Chan, & Shum, 2011; Riggs et al., 2006). Children who are better able to maintain and follow rule sets on measures such as the DCCS are probably better able to control impulsive aggression while understanding and abiding by rules in the different contexts of their lives. Relatedly, parenting characterized by warmth and structure supports developing self-regulation and prosocial conduct. Within positive parent–child relationships, children internalize expectations for appropriate behavior and a sense of self-worth balanced with empathy for others (McKee, Colletti, Rakow, Jones, & Forehand, 2008; Zhou et al., 2002). These adaptive systems also work in concert; EF has been shown to mediate the link between parenting and child externalizing problems in contexts of homelessness and more generally (Piehler et al., 2014; Sulik, Blair, Mills-Koonce, Berry, & Greenberg, 2015).

Contrary to expectations in this study, however, parenting warmth was not associated with child-reported traumatic stress or depression symptoms, and EF was *positively* associated with traumatic stress and depression such that children who performed better on the EF task reported more internalizing symptoms one month later. The lack of association with parenting warmth could be tied to the findings discussed previously, showing that parents underestimated the level of their children's internalizing and traumatic stress symptoms. It could be that, even in the context of a close relationship, some children either feel that their parents do not understand their distress or perceive a need to protect their parents by concealing distress. The ability to mask their negative emotions also could reflect higher EF. Studies with youth in the broader literature have found inconsistent links between EF and internalizing problems, particularly in contexts of stress (Gulley, Hankin, & Young, 2015; Wagner et al., 2015). Some children with good EF and warm parents may be in the more acute phase of adaptation and not yet showing evidence of recovery from the adversity related to their homeless episode. Alternatively, it could be that aspects of the parent–child relationship other than warmth, such as structure and appropriate discipline, would relate to children's traumatic stress and internalizing symptoms.

Summary and Implications

Of course, these findings should be interpreted with caution as they represent a small sample and consider adaptation over a rather short period of just one month. As noted above, it is entirely possible that different trajectories of adjustment and recovery would emerge given more time and more statistical power to compare meaningful subgroups of children, such as those who appear resilient, primarily internalizing, primarily externalizing, and both internalizing and externalizing at the initial time point along with different patterns of competence and problems over time (e.g., Bonanno & Diminich, 2013). While we identified children within our sample who appeared resilient at T1 and T2, with some changing status across the time points, our small sample precluded detailed group comparisons. Person-focused analyses that consider individuals more holistically hold potential for further elucidating trajectories of functioning and how protective factors may influence adaptation (Huntington et al., 2008).

More precise information regarding adaptation to the shelter context could be gleaned with a sample of families all recruited either before or just after their move to emergency housing. This was not possible in the current study due to long stays and little turnover in the family shelter population in this particular municipality, which resulted in substantial variability in the length of time in shelter at T1. Identifying families before their move to emergency housing would be particularly challenging, but with sufficient time and access, identifying families within their first week in emergency housing is feasible. Other limitations of this study include a lack of measures of externalizing problems based on child self-report or other-report, such as teachers or other adults who would know the children well. Clearly it is important in this context, as in others, to consider multiple perspectives on child functioning whenever possible.

Future efforts can aim to follow families and assess parent and child functioning over longer spans of time, including after they move out of emergency housing to more permanent living situations. Increasing our understanding of the adaptive processes leading to resilience in children and families will continue to inform efforts to improve outcomes for all children who experience homelessness. Our findings suggest that children and families are adapting in the context of emergency housing, but that individuals likely differ in their trajectories and durations of adaptation. As such, assessments of child and family functioning in the context of emergency housing would benefit from careful consideration of assessment timing, the possibility of repeating assessments to gauge change, the sources of information beyond parent report, and the likelihood that a good number of families are already rallying their strengths to bounce back despite temporary struggles and setbacks. Developing assessment tools and strategies that can differentiate these families from those unlikely to succeed without more intensive interventions will lead to more efficient, effective policies and practices.

References

Anooshian, L. J. (2005). Violence and aggression in the lives of homeless children: A review. *Aggression and Violent Behavior*, *10*, 129–152. doi:10.1016/j.avb.2003.10.004.

Bassuk, E. L., DeCandia, C. J., Beach, C. A., & Berman, F. (2014). *America's youngest outcasts: A report card on child homelessness*. Waltham, MA: The National Center on Family Homelessness at American Institutes for Research.

Bassuk, E. L., Richard, M. K., & Tsertsvadze, A. (2015). The prevalence of mental illness in homeless children: A systematic review and meta-analysis. *Journal of the American Academy of Child & Adolescent Psychiatry*, *54*, 86–96. doi:10.1016/j.jaac.2014.11.008.

Bassuk, E. L., Volk, K. T., & Olivet, J. (2010). A framework for developing supports and services for families experiencing homelessness. *Open Health Services and Policy Journal*, *3*, 34–40.

Bernier, A., Carlson, S. M., & Whipple, N. (2010). From external regulation to self-regulation: Early parenting precursors of young children's executive functioning. *Child Development*, *81*, 326–339. doi:10.1111/j.1467-8624.2009.01397.x.

Best, J. R., & Miller, P. (2010). A developmental perspective on executive function. *Child Development*, *81*, 1641–1660. doi:10.1111/j.1467-8624.2010.01499.x.

Bonanno, G. A., & Diminich, E. D. (2013). Annual research review: Positive adjustment to adversity—trajectories of minimal-impact resilience and emergent resilience. *Journal of Child Psychology and Psychiatry*, *54*, 378–401. doi:10.1111/jcpp.12021.

Bourdon, K. H., Goodman, R., Rae, D. S., Simpson, G., & Koretz, D. S. (2005). The Strengths and Difficulties Questionnaire: US normative data and psychometric properties. *Journal of the American Academy of Child & Adolescent Psychiatry*, *44*, 557–564. doi:10.1097/01.chi.0000159157.57075.c8.

Buckner, J. C. (2008). Understanding the impact of homelessness on children: Challenges and future research directions. *American Behavioral Scientist*, *51*, 721–736. doi:10.1177/0002764207311984.

Buckner, J. C., Mezzacappa, E., & Beardslee, W. R. (2003). Characteristics of resilient youths living in poverty: The role of self-regulatory processes. Development and Psychopathology, 15, 139–162. doi:10.1017.S0954579403000087

Buckner, J. C., Mezzacappa, E., & Beardslee, W. R. (2009). Self-regulation and its relations to adaptive functioning in low income youths. *American Journal of Orthopsychiatry*, *79*, 19–30. doi:10.1037/a0014796.

Calkins, S. D., & Hill, A. (2007). Caregiver influences on emerging emotion regulation: Biological and environmental transactions in early development. In J. J. Gross (Ed.), *Handbook of emotion regulation* (pp. 229–248). New York: Guilford Press.

Caspi, A., Moffitt, T. E., Morgan, J., Rutter, M., Taylor, A., Arseneault, L., … Polo-Thomas, M. (2004). Maternal expressed emotion predicts children's antisocial behavior problems: Using monozygotic-twin differences to identify environmental effects on behavioral development. *Developmental Psychology*, *40*, 149–161. doi:10.1037/0012-1649.40.2.149.

Cowan, B. (2014). Trauma exposures and mental health outcomes among sheltered children and youth ages 6–18. In M. Haskett, S. Perlman, & B. Cowan (Eds.), *Supporting families experiencing homelessness: Current practices and future directions*. New York: Springer. doi:10.1007/978-1-4614-8718-0_10.

Cutuli, J. J., & Herbers, J. E. (2014). Promoting resilience for children who experience family homelessness: Opportunities to encourage developmental competence. *Cityscape*, *16*, 113–139.

Cutuli, J. J., Desjardins, C. D., Herbers, J. E., Long, J. D., Heistad, D., Chan, C. K., … Masten, A. S. (2013). Academic achievement trajectories of homeless and highly mobile students: Resilience in the context of chronic and acute risk. *Child Development*, *84*, 841–857. doi:10.1111/cdev.12013.

Cutuli, J. J., Herbers, J. E., Masten, A. S., & Reed, M. (in press). Resilience in development. In C. R. Snyder & S. J. Lopez (Eds.), *The handbook of positive psychology* (3rd ed.).

DePrince, A. P., Weinzierl, K. M., & Combs, M. D. (2009). Executive function performance and trauma exposure in a community sample of children. *Child Abuse & Neglect, 33*, 353–361. doi:10.1016/j.chiabu.2008.08.002.
Derogatis, L. R., Lipman, R. S., Rickels, K., Uhlenhuth, E. H., & Covi, L. (1974). The Hopkins Symptom Checklist (HSCL): A self-report symptom inventory. *Behavioral Science, 19*, 1–15. doi:10.1002/bs.3830190102.
Diamond, A., & Lee, K. (2011). Interventions shown to aid executive function development in children 4 to 12 years old. *Science, 333*(6045), 959–964. doi:10.1126/science.1204529.
Garon, N., Bryson, S. E., & Smith, I. M. (2008). Executive function in preschoolers: A review using an integrative framework. *Psychological Bulletin, 134*, 31–60. doi:10.1037/0033-2909.134.1.31.
Goodman, R. (1997). The strengths and difficulties questionnaire: A research note. *Journal of Child Psychology and Psychiatry, 38*, 581–586. doi:10.1111/j.1469-7610.1997.tb01545.x.
Gulley, L. D., Hankin, B. L., & Young, J. F. (2015). Risk for depression and anxiety in youth: The interaction between negative affectivity, effortful control, and stressors. *Journal of Abnormal Child Psychology, 44*, 207–218. doi:10.1007/s10802-015-9997-7.
Haskett, M. E., Armstrong, J. M., & Tisdale, J. (2015). Developmental status and social-emotional functioning of young children experiencing homelessness. *Early Childhood Education Journal, 44*, 119–125. doi:10.1007/s10643-015-0691-8.
Herbers, J. E., Cutuli, J. J., Lafavor, T. L., Vrieze, D., Leibel, C., Obradovic, J., & Masten, A. S. (2011). Direct and indirect effects of parenting on academic functioning of young homeless children. *Early Education and Development, 22*, 77–104. doi:10.1080/10409280903507261.
Herbers, J. E., Cutuli, J. J., Supkoff, L. S., Narayan, A. J., & Masten, A. S. (2014). Parenting and co-regulation: Adaptive systems for competence in children experiencing homelessness. *American Journal of Orthopsychiatry, 84*, 420–430. doi:10.1037/h0099843.
Hughes, C., & Ensor, R. (2011). Individual differences in growth in executive function across the transition to school predict externalizing and internalizing behaviors and self-perceived academic success at 6 years of age. *Journal of Experimental Child Psychology, 108*, 663–676. doi:10.1016/j.jecp.2010.06.005.
Huntington, N., Buckner, J. C., & Bassuk, E. L. (2008). Adaptation in homeless children: An empirical examination using cluster analysis. *American Behavioral Scientist, 51*, 737–755. doi:10.1177/0002764207311985.
Kassam-Adams, N., Garcia-Espana, J. F., Miller, V. A., & Winston, F. (2006). Parent-child agreement regarding children's acute stress: The role of parent acute stress reactions. *Journal of the American Academy of Child and Adolescent Psychiatry, 45*, 1485–1493. doi:10.1097/01.chi.0000237703.97518.12.
Kisiel, C., Conradi, L., Fehrenbach, T., Torgersen, E., & Briggs, E. C. (2014). Assessing the effects of trauma in children and adolescents in practice settings. *Child and Adolescent Psychiatric Clinics of North America, 23*, 223–242.
Kovacs, M. (2003). *Children's depression inventory technical manual update*. Toronto, ON: Multi-Health Systems.
Kovacs, M. (2011). *Children's depression inventory 2nd edition technical manual*. Toronto, ON: Multi-Health Systems.
Luthar, S. S., & Brown, P. J. (2007). Maximizing resilience through diverse levels of inquiry: Prevailing paradigms, possibilities, and priorities for the future. *Development and Psychopathology, 19*, 931–955. doi:10.1017/S0954579407000454.
Luthar, S. S., Crossman, E. J., & Small, P. J. (2015). Resilience and adversity. In R. M. Lerner, M. H. Bornstein, & T. Leventhal (Eds.), *Handbook of child psychology and developmental science* (7th ed., Vol. 3, pp. 247–286). New York: Wiley.
Magana, A. B., Goldstein, M. J., Karno, M., Miklowitz, D. J., Jenkins, J., & Falloon, I. R. H. (1986). A brief method for assessing expressed emotion in relatives of psychiatric patients. *Psychiatry Research, 17*, 203–212. doi:10.1016/0165-1781(86)90049-1.

Masten, A. S. (2001). Ordinary magic: Resilience processes in development. *American Psychologist, 56*(3), 227–238. doi:10.1037/0003-066X.56.3.227.

Masten, A. S. (2014). *Ordinary magic: Resilience in development*. New York: Guilford Publications.

Masten, A. S., & Cicchetti, D. (in press). Resilience in development: Progress and transformation. In D. Cicchetti (Ed.), *Developmental psychopathology* (3rd ed., Vol. IV). New York, NY: Routledge.

Masten, A. S., Cutuli, J. J., Herbers, J. E., Hinz, E., Obradovic, J., & Wenzel, A. J. (2014). Academic risk and resilience in the context of homelessness. *Child Development Perspectives, 8*, 201–206. doi:10.1111/cdep.12088.

Masten, A. S., Herbers, J. E., Desjardins, C. D., Cutuli, J. J., McCormick, C. M., Sapienza, J. K., . . . Zelazo, P. D. (2012). Executive function skills and school success in young children experiencing homelessness. *Educational Researcher, 41*(9), 375–384. doi:10.3102/0013189X12459883.

Masten, A. S., Miliotis, D., Graham-Bermann, S. A., Ramirez, M. L., & Neemann, J. (1993). Children in homeless families: Risks to mental health and development. *Journal of Consulting and Clinical Psychology, 61*, 335–343.

McKee, L., Colletti, C., Rakow, A., Jones, D. J., & Forehand, R. (2008). Parenting and child externalizing behaviors: Are the associations specific or diffuse? *Aggression and Violence, 13*, 201–215. doi:10.1016/j.avb.2008.03.005.

Meiser-Stedman, R., Smith, P., Glucksman, E., Yule, W., & Dalgleish, T. (2007). Parent and child agreement for acute stress disorder, post-traumatic stress disorder and other psychopathology in a prospective study of children and adolescents exposed to single-event trauma. *Journal of Abnormal Child Psychology, 35*, 191–201. doi:10.1007/s10802-006-9068-1.

Narayan, A. J., Herbers, J. E., Plowman, E. J., Gewirtz, A. H., & Masten, A. S. (2012). Expressed emotion in homeless families: A methodological study of the Five-Minute Speech Sample. *Journal of Family Psychology, 26*, 648–653. doi:10.1037/a0028968.

National-Institute-of-Health (2011). *NIH Toolbox: Assessment of neurological and behavioral function*. Retrieved March 7, 2011, from http://www.nihtoolbox.org/WebPart%20Pages/Cognition.aspx

Obradovic, J. (2010). Effortful control and adaptive functioning of homeless children: Variable-focused and person-focused analyses. *Journal of Applied Developmental Psychology, 31*, 109–117. doi:10.1016/j.appdev.2009.09.004.

Ogilvie, J. M., Stewart, A. L., Chan, R. C. K., & Shum, D. H. K. (2011). Neuropsychological measures of executive function and antisocial behavior: A meta-analysis. *Criminology, 49*, 1063–1107. doi:10.1111/j.1745-9125.2011.00252.x.

Perlman, S., Cowan, B., Gewirtz, A., Haskett, M., & Stokes, L. (2012). Promoting positive parenting in the context of homelessness. *American Journal of Orthopsychiatry, 82*, 402–412. doi:10.1111/j.1939-0025.2012.01158.x.

Piehler, T. F., Bloomquist, M. L., August, G. J., Gewirtz, A. H., Lee, S. S., & Lee, W. S. (2014). Executive functioning as a mediator of conduct problems prevention in children of homeless families residing in temporary supportive housing: A parallel process latent growth modeling approach. *Journal of Abnormal Child Psychology, 42*, 681–692. doi:10.1007/s10802-013-9816-y.

Pynoos, R., Rodriguez, N., Steinberg, A., Stuber, M., & Frederick, C. (1998). *The UCLA PTSD reaction index for DSM IV (revision 1)*. Los Angeles: UCLA Trauma Psychiatry Program.

Rafferty, Y., Shinn, M., & Weitzman, B. C. (2004). Academic achievement among formerly homeless adolescents and their continuously housed peers. *Journal of School Psychology, 42* (3), 179–199. doi:10.1016/j.jsp.2004.02.002.

Riggs, N. R., Jahromi, L. B., Razza, R. P., Dillworth-Bart, J. E., & Mueller, U. (2006). Executive function and the promotion of social-emotional competence. *Journal of Applied Developmental Psychology, 27*, 300–309. doi:10.1016/j.appdev.2006.04.002.

Rubin, D. B. (1987). *Multiple imputation for nonresponse in surveys*. New York: Wiley.

Rutter, M. (2013). Annual research review: Resilience: Clinical implications. *Journal of Child Psychology and Psychiatry, 54*, 474–487. doi:10.1111/j.1469-7610.2012.02615.x.

Samuels, J., Shinn, M., & Buckner, J. C. (2010). *Homeless children: Update on research, policy, programs, and opportunities*. Prepared for the Office of the Assistant Secretary for Planning and Evaluation, U.S. Department of Health and Human Services.

Sandanger, I., Moum, T., Ingebrigtsen, G., Dalgard, O. S., Sorensen, T., & Bruusgaard, D. (1998). Concordance between symptom screening and diagnostic procedure: The Hopkins Symptom Checklist-25 and the Composite International Diagnostic Interview I. *Social Psychiatry and Psychiatric Epidemiology*, *33*, 345–354. doi:10.1007/s001270050064.

Schafer, J. L., & Graham, J. W. (2002). Missing data: Our view of the state of the art. *Psychological Methods*, *7*, 147–177. doi:10.1177/0049124102030003008.

Schneider, W., Eschman, A., & Zuccolotto, A. (2012). *E-Prime user's guide*. Pittsburgh: Psychology Software Tools.

Shemesh, E., Newcorn, J. H., Rockmore, L., Shneider, B. L., Emre, S., Gelb, B. D., . . . Yehuda, R. (2005). Comparison of parent and child reports of emotional trauma symptoms in pediatric outpatient settings. *Pediatrics*, *115*, e582–e589. doi:10.1542/peds.2004-2201.

Sher-Censor, E. (2015). Five Minute Speech Sample in developmental research: A review. *Developmental Review*, *36*, 127–155. doi:10.1016/j.dr.2015.01.005.

Shinn, M., Schteingart, J. S., Williams, N. C., Carlin-Mathis, J., Bialo-Karagis, N., Becker-Klein, R., & Weitzman, B. C. (2008). Long-term associations of homelessness with children's well-being. *American Behavioral Scientist*, *51*, 789–809. doi:10.1177/0002764207311988.

Snyder, H. R., Miyake, A., & Hankin, B. L. (2015). Advancing understanding of executive function impairments and psychopathology: Bridging the gap between clinical and cognitive approaches. *Frontiers in Psychology*, *6*, 328–342. doi:10.3389/fpsyg.2015.00328.

Southwick, S. M., Bonanno, G. A., Masten, A. S., Panter-Brick, C., & Yehuda, R. (2014). Resilience definitions, theory, and challenges: Interdisciplinary perspectives. *European Journal of Psychotraumatology*, *5*, 25338. doi:10.3402/ejpt.v5.25338.

Stover, C. S., Hahn, H., Berkowitz, S., & Im, J. J. Y. (2010). Agreement of parent and child reports of trauma exposure and symptoms in the early aftermath of a traumatic event. *Psychological Trauma: Theory, Research, Practice, and Policy*, *2*, 159–168. doi:10.1037/a0019156.

Sulik, M. J., Blair, C., Mills-Koonce, R., Berry, D., & Greenberg, M. (2015). Early parenting and the development of externalizing behavior problems: Longitudinal mediation through children's executive function. *Child Development*, *86*, 1588–1603. doi:10.1111/cdev.12386.

Wagner, C. A., Alloy, L. B., & Abramson, L. Y. (2015). Trait rumination, depression, and executive functions in early adolescence. *Journal of Youth and Adolescence*, *44*, 18–36. doi:10.1007/s10964-014-0133-8.

Wechsler, D. (2003). *WISC-IV: Administration and scoring manual*. San Antonio: Psychological Corporation.

Wechsler, D., & Hsiao-pin, C. (2011). *WASI-II: Wechsler abbreviated scale of intelligence*. San Antonio: Pearson.

Zelazo, P. D. (2006). The Dimensional Change Card Sort (DCCS): A method of assessing executive function in children. *Nature Protocols*, *1*, 297–301. doi:10.1038/nprot.2006.46.

Zelazo, P. D., Anderson, J. E., & Richler, J. (2011). *Validation of the NIH toolbox: Executive function, working memory, and sustained attention*. Paper presented at the biennial meeting of the Society for Research on Child Development Montreal, QC, Canada.

Zhou, Q., Eisenberg, N., Losoya, S. H., Fabes, R. A., Reiser, M., Guthrie, I. K., . . . Shepard, S. A. (2002). The relations of parental warmth and positive expressiveness to children's empathy-related responding and social functioning: A longitudinal study. *Child Development*, *73*, 893–915. doi:10.1111/1467-8624.00446.

Chapter 3
Observed Parenting in Families Exposed to Homelessness: Child and Parent Characteristics as Predictors of Response to the Early Risers Intervention

Kendal Holtrop, Timothy F. Piehler, Abigail H. Gewirtz, and Gerald J. August

Introduction

Positive parenting is one of the most important mechanisms capable of protecting children from threats to healthy development posed by homelessness (Cutuli & Herbers, 2014). While it is important to recognize that parents who are homeless can still be committed to their parenting role and maintain positive parenting practices (Gewirtz, DeGarmo, Plowman, August, & Realmuto, 2009; Holtrop, McNeil, & McWey, 2015), experiencing homelessness exposes parents to a host of risk factors that can erode effective caregiving (Cutuli & Herbers, 2014).

Homeless parents report a number of life stressors which have been associated with negative parenting (Torquati, 2002). Individuals experiencing homelessness are also at risk for acute trauma exposure. Homeless women face high rates of

---

Author Note: Kendal Holtrop, Department of Family and Child Sciences, Florida State University; Timothy F. Piehler, Department of Family Social Science, University of Minnesota; Abigail H. Gewirtz, Department of Family Social Science and Institute of Child Development, University of Minnesota; Gerald J. August, Department of Family Social Science, University of Minnesota.This study was funded in part by grant number R01MH074610 from NIMH to Gerald August. We acknowledge with gratitude the families who participated in the Early Risers prevention trial and the participating agencies for their valuable partnership and work to support formerly homeless children and families.

K. Holtrop (✉)
Department of Family and Child Sciences, Florida State University,
208 Sandels Building, Tallahassee, FL 32306, USA
e-mail: kholtrop@fsu.edu

T.F. Piehler • G.J. August
Department of Family Social Science, University of Minnesota, St. Paul, MN, USA

A.H. Gewirtz
Department of Family Social Science and Institute of Child Development,
University of Minnesota, St. Paul, MN, USA

M.E. Haskett (ed.), *Child and Family Well-Being and Homelessness*,
SpringerBriefs in Psychology, DOI 10.1007/978-3-319-50886-3_3

physical and sexual victimization (Arangua, Andersen, & Gelberg, 2005) that exceed those of impoverished, housed women (Rayburn et al., 2005). Homeless men also report extensive trauma histories (Kim, Ford, Howard, & Bradford, 2010). Experiencing trauma can present many risks to parenting (Appleyard & Osofsky, 2003), and among homeless parents, adulthood trauma may be a risk factor for parent–child separation (Zlotnick, Tam, & Bradley, 2007). Furthermore, homeless women report experiencing significantly less social support and greater levels of conflict than never homeless women (Anderson & Rayens, 2004). These factors in particular have been associated with harsh parenting practices among homeless mothers (Marra et al., 2009). It is clear that parenting is an important intervention target among homeless families (Gewirtz, Burkhart, Loehman, & Haukebo, 2014; Perlman, Cowan, Gewirtz, Haskett, & Stokes, 2012).

Efforts to support positive parenting among homeless families are critical for promoting the mental health and developmental needs of children exposed to homelessness. Among homeless and formerly homeless families, positive parenting behaviors have been associated with better child adjustment and may serve as protective factors (Gewirtz et al., 2009; McNeil Smith, Holtrop, & Reynolds, 2015). Fortunately, there have been a number of recent efforts to develop and implement interventions with the goal of improving parenting practices and child outcomes among homeless families (see Gewirtz, 2007; Haskett, Loehman, & Burkhart, 2016; Perlman et al., 2012). While these efforts appear promising (e.g., Gewirtz & Taylor, 2009; Perlman et al., 2012), the empirical research examining these interventions is still underdeveloped (Gewirtz et al., 2014; Haskett et al., 2016). Specifically, there is a need for further research utilizing larger sample sizes, control groups, and more sophisticated measurement strategies (Haskett et al., 2016). It is also critical to attend to the substantial heterogeneity in characteristics and needs among homeless families when providing and evaluating interventions (Herbers & Cutuli, 2014; Perlman et al., 2012). In this regard, examining moderation can help explain variability in treatment response and offer insight about the subpopulations most likely to benefit from an intervention. This could provide important data for tailoring interventions to diverse homeless populations and enhancing the clinical impact and cost-effectiveness of intervention efforts. Accordingly, the aim of the current study was to identify parent and child characteristics among families exposed to homelessness that differentially predict changes in parenting in response to a psychosocial preventive intervention.

Focal Intervention: The Early Risers Program

The Early Risers program is a preventive intervention that seeks to avert the development of conduct disorders and substance abuse among high-risk children (August, Realmuto, Hektner, & Bloomquist, 2001; August, Realmuto, Winters, & Hektner, 2001). The program includes both a child and family/parent component to promote skill development in multiple domains. The intervention component meant to strengthen parenting skills draws on social learning theory, with the goal of teaching parents behavioral management strategies that can interrupt coercive family processes and ultimately improve child compliance (August, Realmuto, Hektner, et al., 2001). Longitudinal investigations of the Early Risers program have confirmed changes in parenting practices play an important mediational role in promoting positive child behavioral outcomes (e.g., Hektner, August, Bloomquist, Lee, & Klimes-Dougan, 2014). Efforts to better understand changes in parenting practices resulting from the Early Risers intervention, therefore, constitute a valuable area for further exploration.

A strength of the Early Risers intervention is that it has been implemented and evaluated in a variety of contexts (e.g., August, Lee, Bloomquist, Realmuto, & Hektner, 2003; August, Realmuto, Hektner, et al., 2001). The current study will examine findings from a cluster randomized effectiveness trial among formerly homeless families living in a number of supportive housing agencies. Outcome data indicate the Early Risers intervention was successful at improving parent self-efficacy and reducing parent reports of child depression 2 years post-baseline. Improvement in parent self-efficacy was also found to predict effective observed parenting, which in turn was associated with better child adjustment (Gewirtz, DeGarmo, Lee, Morrell, & August, 2015). At 3 years post-baseline, participation in the Early Risers intervention was associated with reduced growth in child conduct problems. Child executive functioning was found to fully mediate these improvements (Piehler, Bloomquist, et al., 2014). However, no main effect of the Early Risers intervention was found on parenting practices (Gewirtz et al., 2015). The impetus behind the current study is to extend our understanding beyond main effects of the intervention condition to an examination of predictors of variability in intervention response.

Predictors of Intervention Response

Child behavior problems. In contrast to earlier reports suggesting increased behavior problem severity is linked to poor treatment response (e.g., Assemany & McIntosh, 2002), meta-analytic studies indicate higher levels of initial child problem behavior are associated with greater effect sizes for child behavioral outcomes (Lundahl, Risser, & Lovejoy, 2006; Menting, Orobio de Castro, & Matthys, 2013). A significant moderation effect, however, was not evidenced in at least one recent study (Gardner, Hutchings, Bywater, & Whitaker, 2010). Specific to the Early Risers intervention, pretreatment levels of child aggression have been found to differentially predict child outcomes over time, with treatment outcomes at follow-up favoring the more severely aggressive children (August, Hektner, Egan, Realmuto, & Bloomquist, 2002; August et al., 2003). Less research has examined parenting practice outcomes. Meta-analytic results suggest baseline level of child behavior problems may not significantly influence intervention impact on parenting (Lundahl et al., 2006; Nowak & Heinrichs, 2008). Yet, Chamberlain et al. (2008)

found parents in their intervention group significantly improved on positive reinforcement only when their child had more behavior problems; this change was not evident among parents of children with fewer behavior problems, indicating a moderator effect. In Early Risers research, child behavior problems have been implicated in a complex interaction with intervention dosage to affect parental distress but not discipline practices (August et al., 2002; August, Realmuto, Hektner, et al., 2001).

Parental depression. Maternal depression has generally been associated with poorer treatment response in studies examining child behavioral outcomes (Reyno & McGrath, 2006). When investigated in the presence of a control group, maternal depression has been implicated as a significant moderator of treatment effect on child behavior (Gardner et al., 2010). In this case, mothers with a higher level of depression reported better child outcomes in the intervention condition compared to the control condition; this difference was largely due to depressed mothers in the control condition reporting particularly poor child outcomes. However, not all studies have found evidence of moderation (van den Hoofdakker et al., 2010). The literature examining the effect of parental depression on parenting practice outcomes is limited. Baydar, Reid, and Webster-Stratton (2003) found similar patterns of change in parenting among intervention attenders regardless of high or low depressive symptoms. In a study of moderators of coercive parenting, McTaggart and Sanders (2007) did not find a significant interaction between parental depression and intervention group status. Yet, related research on Early Risers found parental well-being moderated parenting efficacy outcomes in response to intervention delivery method (Piehler, Lee, Bloomquist, & August, 2014), suggesting a continued need to investigate the influence of parental depression.

Parenting self-efficacy. In a study of the association between parenting self-efficacy and intervention outcomes, higher parenting self-efficacy was found to be significantly associated with better intervention-specific parenting scores for mothers; a similar, although marginally significant, association was found for fathers (Spoth, Redmond, Haggerty, & Ward, 1995). Beyond these predictive effects, investigations examining the role of parenting self-efficacy have suggested that it may function as a mediator between intervention participation and improvements in parenting practices (McTaggart & Sanders, 2007), child outcomes (O'Connor, Rodriguez, Cappella, Morris, & McClowry, 2012; but see Gardner, Burton, & Klimes, 2006), or both (Gewirtz et al., 2015). Efforts to test parenting self-efficacy as a moderator of treatment outcome have generally not found support (McTaggart & Sanders, 2007; Spoth et al., 1995). However, maternal self-efficacy was found to moderate treatment response in a study of children with attention deficit/hyperactivity disorder (ADHD; van den Hoofdakker et al., 2010). That study examined child and parent variables influencing the effectiveness of adding a parent training component to routine clinical care for ADHD, as compared to routine clinical care alone. Results showed that adding the parent training component resulted in superior child outcomes, but only among families with higher parenting self-efficacy. Recent findings have also highlighted the role of parenting self-efficacy within the Early Risers intervention (Gewirtz et al., 2015; Piehler, Lee, et al., 2014), suggesting an opportunity for further research.

Parent–child attachment. The bulk of research investigating the influence of attachment on child and parent intervention outcomes has focused on assessing general parental attachment, as opposed to parent–child attachment, and has evaluated programs targeting the early parent–child relationship. In an intervention for couples experiencing the transition to parenthood, parent reports of attachment insecurity in close relationships moderated intervention effects, with individual and family outcomes showing greater benefit in situations where parents—especially fathers—had poor initial attachment scores (Feinberg & Kan, 2008). In contrast, a study of the effects of Early Head Start on parenting practices showed an opposite pattern; program mothers demonstrated more favorable effects when they had better self-reported initial attachment scores with people emotionally close to them (Berlin et al., 2011). Other findings have been disparate and suggest maternal self-reported attachment may interact with depression to differentially predict intervention outcomes within home visiting programs (Duggan, Berlin, Cassidy, Burrell, & Tandon, 2009; Robinson & Emde, 2004). Further research is needed to determine how attachment, particularly parent–child attachment, influences intervention outcomes and to evaluate programs targeting families of school-age children, such as Early Risers.

Purpose of the Study

The literature examining predictors of child and parent intervention outcomes and moderators of treatment response is limited and largely inconclusive. Further research is needed to determine which characteristics differentially predict parenting practice outcomes following participation in psychosocial preventive interventions. The purpose of this study was to identify which child and parent characteristics predict differential responses to the Early Risers intervention among formerly homeless families residing in supportive housing. We chose to examine changes in parenting practices as our focal outcome because of the importance ascribed to positive parenting within Early Risers as well as among families exposed to homelessness. In this study, the parenting practice variable was derived from repeated, observational assessment of ineffective discipline practices measured across four waves of data collection, which constitutes a key study strength and contribution to the literature on parenting and homeless families. We hypothesized that child behavior problems, parental depression, parenting self-efficacy, and parent–child attachment would each function as moderators influencing the effect of the Early Risers intervention on change in observed ineffective discipline practices. Given the disparate findings in previous research investigating these moderators, we chose not to make specific predictions about the directionality of the effects. The results of this study have the potential to advance understanding of variability in response to treatment among subgroups of homeless families and inform future efforts to optimize impact of the Early Risers intervention on parenting practices.

Methods

Intervention Sites

Through a community–university collaboration dedicated to helping children and families exposed to homelessness (the Healthy Families Network; Gewirtz, 2007), a randomized effectiveness trial of the Early Risers intervention was conducted across 16 private, nonprofit supportive housing agencies in a large metropolitan area of the Midwest. These agencies serve more than 95% of the single-site family supportive housing population in the area. To qualify for supportive housing, families had to be homeless at the time of admission. In addition, most sites required families to demonstrate additional burden, such as caregiver mental illness, substance use, or the need to evade domestic violence. The 16 housing sites were randomly assigned to either the intervention condition or treatment as usual. Usual services varied somewhat across sites, but typically included case management, education and/or job training, and access to medical services. Some sites also offered childcare or after-school activities.

Participants

To be eligible for the current study, parents had to reside at one of 16 participating supportive housing sites and be living with at least one child between 6–12 years old. Initial enrollment included 161 parents with 270 children. One of the housing sites did not have any eligible participants and was dropped from the study. After enrolling in the study, but prior to providing baseline data, some families relocated or dropped out of the study. More detailed information about the recruitment process and participant retention is reported by Gewirtz et al. (2015). The current study utilized data from four assessment points and includes a sample of 137 parents with 223 children from 15 supportive housing sites. The study sample included all single-headed families; in the vast majority of cases (98.5%) families were headed by a female. Almost half (48%) of the parents in the sample were African American, 21% were multiracial, 19% were Caucasian, and 12% were from other racial/ethnic groups. Average annual parent income was \$10,457.22 (SD = \$5594.65). Parents had the equivalent of about a high school education ($M = 12.00$ years of education; SD = 1.66). Among the children in the study, the mean child age was 8.12 years (SD = 2.3). The gender dispersal was fairly even (49% girls). The majority (68%) of children also had a sibling in the study, and the number of children per family ranged from 1 to 5, with a mean of 1.6 children per family. The number of families participating in the study at each different supportive housing site varied from 1 to 34; an average of 14.87 children participated per site. Study families had moved an average of 1.4 times (SD = 1.4) in the year prior to baseline enrollment, and 18.5% of families had moved three or more times that year. As many as one-third (34%) of the children were part of an open child protection case at the baseline assessment.

Intervention

Early Risers is an evidence-based, multicomponent preventive intervention that targets risk factors at various ecological levels (e.g., child competence, family interactions, peer influence, community context) and works to build child and parent competencies that promote positive outcomes. In this study, intervention programming was delivered over the course of 2 years. The child component consisted of skills-focused education and behavioral intervention meant to improve academic success, emotion regulation, and interpersonal competence. This took place through an after-school program held during the school year and a 6-week camp offered during the summers. The child component utilized the Promoting Alternative Thinking Strategies (PATHS) curriculum (Kusché & Greenberg, 1994) along with a literacy enhancement component. The parenting skills component included two different elements. The first year of programming offered "family fun nights" which provided opportunities for positive parent–child interaction combined with information on child development. During the second year, parents participated in the evidence-based Parenting Through Change program (PTC; Forgatch & DeGarmo, 1999). The goal of PTC is to help parents improve five core parenting practices: skill encouragement, discipline, monitoring, problem solving, and positive involvement. In addition, the Early Risers intervention integrated a family support component in which participants received access to family support (i.e., case management) services on an individualized basis. Fidelity to the Early Risers program and its associated intervention components (i.e., PATHS, PTC) was confirmed using observational measures. Further information about the intervention, including the fidelity assessment process, is reported elsewhere (Gewirtz et al., 2015).

Interventionists

The Early Risers intervention was delivered by family advocates. Each family advocate had prior experience providing case management or advocacy services to homeless families and had a bachelor's degree or at least some relevant higher education. Advocates were each in charge of providing services at two housing sites. Approximately 40 h of initial training was provided to the advocates in the overall Early Risers intervention as well as in specific aspects of PATHS and PTC. Advocates also received ongoing coaching through weekly meetings with the Early Risers program manager.

Assessment Procedures

Prior to beginning assessments, written consent was received from participants in accordance with the procedures approved by the Institutional Review Board. Research assistants met with participants in their home in order to complete assessments, either on-site at the supportive housing agency or off-site if the family had transitioned to other housing. The parent and target child both participated in the assessment process. In families where more than one child participated in the study, individual assessment sessions were conducted with each parent and child. Each parent received a $50 gift card for their participation in the assessment. Assessments were conducted at four time points: at baseline (T0), after 1 year of intervention (T1), after 2 years of intervention (T2), and at 1-year follow-up post-intervention (T3).

Measures

Demographic covariates. Information regarding parent race/ethnicity, parent education, child age, and child gender was gathered during a structured interview conducted with parents during baseline data collection.

Parenting practices. Parenting practices were evaluated through observational ratings of parent–child interaction during structured Family Interaction Tasks (FITs). In the current study, the FITs protocol lasted approximately 20 min and included the following four activities: (a) a dyadic problem solving task, (b) a guessing game, (c) a labyrinth game, and (d) a "tangoes" puzzle activity. Families were debriefed upon completion to address any questions or concerns.

The FITs assessments were videotaped and coded using established ratings of key parenting practices (DeGarmo, Patterson, & Forgatch, 2004). Trained coders, blind to intervention condition, viewed the tapes and rated parent and child behavior during each of the four activities according to a four-point scale ranging from *Hardly Ever Applies* to *Applies All of the Time*. Reliability checks were performed by evaluating interrater reliability among a randomly selected subset of tapes (24 %). The overall FITs protocol and coding procedure has been described elsewhere in more detail (Gewirtz et al., 2009; Gewirtz et al., 2015).

For the current study, an ineffective discipline score was derived as the focal outcome for the parenting practices variable. The score was computed using 11 items reflecting observed discipline practices within the FITs, such as "Overly strict, authoritarian, oppressive," "Expresses anger/hostility when disciplining," "Uses nagging or nattering to get compliance," "Threatens or uses physical punishment," and "Erratic, haphazard, inconsistent." Chronbach's alpha for the scale ranged from 0.75 to 0.86 at each wave of assessment. The overall intraclass correlation coefficient (ICC), an index of interrater reliability, was 0.69.

Child behavior problems. Parents completed the Parent Rating Scales of the Behavior Assessment System for Children, Second Edition (BASC-2; Reynolds & Kamphaus, 2004). Child behavior problems were assessed using the 30-item Externalizing Problems composite scale, which measures indicators of aggression, conduct problems, and hyperactivity. Parents indicate the frequency of each child behavior on a four-point scale ranging from *never* (0) to *almost always* (3). T scores were then derived for use in the analyses, with higher scores reflecting greater child behavior problems. The BASC-2 is a well-established assessment with demonstrated psychometric properties (Reynolds & Kamphaus, 2004).

Parental depression. The Brief Symptom Inventory 18 (BSI 18; Derogatis, 2000) was administered to measure parent psychological distress. For this study, the six items designed to assess depression were used to derive a score on the parental depression variable. Parents indicated how distressed they felt by each symptom on a five-point scale ranging from *not at all* (0) to *extremely* (4). Items were then summed and converted to standardized T scores, with higher scores indicating greater depressive symptoms. Use of the BSI 18 has been validated within a variety of populations and contexts (e.g., Prelow, Weaver, Swenson, & Bowman, 2005).

Parenting self-efficacy. Parenting self-efficacy scores were derived from the Parenting Relationship Questionnaire (PRQ; Kamphaus & Reynolds, 2006). This self-report measure assesses multiple domains of parenting and has shown evidence for reliability and validity (Kamphaus & Reynolds, 2006). Specifically, the 8-item Parenting Confidence scale was used to assess feelings of competence and control in the parenting role. Each item was rated on a four-point scale ranging from *never* (0) to *almost always* (3). Items were then summed and converted to standardized T scores, with higher scores indicating greater levels of parenting self-efficacy.

Parent–child attachment. The PRQ (Kamphaus & Reynolds, 2006) was also used to assess parent–child attachment. The 11-item Attachment scale measures various aspects of the parent–child relationship, as reported by the parent, that are associated with emotional responsiveness (e.g., empathy, understanding). Items are rated on a four-point scale ranging from *never* (0) to *almost always* (3). Items were then summed and converted to standardized T scores, with higher scores indicating greater levels of parent–child attachment.

Results

Analytic Strategy

Intent-to-treat analyses were used to examine intervention effects. Latent growth models (LGM) were estimated using the structural equation modeling program Mplus version 7 (Muthén & Muthén, 2012). Growth was modeled over four assessment time points, including baseline, year one, year two (post-intervention), and year three (one-year follow-up). All variables examined in a moderating role were measured at baseline.

The multilevel nature of the dataset was accounted for in all primary analyses. Parent–child dyads (n = 223) represented the primary level of analysis. These dyads were nested within families (n = 137), and families were nested within intervention sites (n = 15). Data from parent–child dyads within a family and shared intervention site are not fully independent and could violate standard assumptions of independence. Note that Mplus does not treat repeated measures on individual subjects as a level of analysis in clustered data (Muthén & Muthén, 2012).

Two approaches were utilized to account for the multilevel nature of the dataset. First, in order to account for the nesting of individual parent–child dyads within families, we used the Mplus "TYPE IS COMPLEX" feature. This feature computes adjusted standard errors of parameters and chi-square tests of model fit to account for multilevel data. It is useful for complex models such as the described LGM. However, the COMPLEX feature is only able to account for single clustering variable and cannot incorporate an additional level of analysis (Muthén & Muthén, 2012). Therefore, the additional level of the dataset (nesting within intervention sites) was accounted for using a more traditional two-level modeling approach (e.g., Duncan et al., 1997) in conjunction with the COMPLEX feature (COMPLEX TWOLEVEL). This required the estimation of all growth models at both the individual parent–child dyad (i.e., within) level and at the site level (i.e., between). Because of the cluster-randomized design, all intervention effects were examined at the site level of analysis. To examine moderation, all interaction effects with intervention condition were computed at the parent–child (within) level.

A stepwise approach was used to test for moderation. First, the slope of the multilevel LGM was regressed on all covariates as main effects (i.e., direct effects), including demographic covariates (i.e., parent race/ethnicity, parent education, child age, child gender), intervention status (i.e., intervention versus control), and child/parent variables (i.e., child problem behaviors, parental depression, parenting self-efficacy, parent–child attachment). All covariates were centered around their means and allowed to covary with the latent intercept in the model, with the exception of intervention status. Following estimation of the main effects model, interaction models were estimated, including interaction terms between intervention status and each parent/child variable. Because of multicollinearity between interaction terms, each interaction term was initially added to the main effects model individually to test for significance. Those interaction terms that achieved significance were retained and added together to a final interaction model. Nonsignificant child/parent predictors were dropped from the model in order to examine the most parsimonious model. All demographic variables were retained in the final model regardless of significance.

Missing values were present in the dataset due to the longitudinal nature of the design, but adequate covariance coverage was present (ranging from 0.51 to 0.96). A missing value analysis was conducted using SPSS software version 22. The Little's MCAR test conducted on all measures included in the models was consistent with values missing completely at random, $\chi 2(108) = 125.64, p = 0.12$. Missing data in all models were managed with the full information maximum likelihood (FIML) procedure used by Mplus version 7. This method has been shown to be very efficient when analyzing data from samples with moderate levels of missing values. When using FIML, the estimation of each parameter is made on the basis of all available information from each participant. Consequently, we can retain participants with missing data in the analysis so they contribute to model estimation.

The fit of each estimated model to the data was evaluated. A good model fit should yield a nonsignificant χ^2 value, but this test often does not provide a complete picture of model fit and other fit indices may be preferred (Kline, 2005). We evaluated fit indices according to Hu and Bentler (1999), who suggest a CFI < 0.95 and an SRMR <0.09 indicate acceptable model fit.

Preliminary Analyses

Table 3.1 includes correlations and descriptive statistics of key study variables. Attrition over the course of the intervention was examined for the two conditions. Attrition was due to loss of families at follow-up or a family's decision to drop out of the study. For the present study, we also considered those families who declined to participate in the FIT at the 1-year follow-up (T3) to have attrited. Over the four assessment points, 223 parent-child dyads provided data, including 215 at baseline. A few participants (often siblings) entered the study after the baseline assessment. At baseline (T0), 155 parent–child dyads completed the FIT, 136 at year one (T1), 118 at year two (T2), and 108 at year three (T3). One-hundred and eighty-five parent–child dyads completed the FIT at some point during at least one of the four assessment points.

An analysis comparing participants who attrited at any point during the study ($n = 115$) with those participants who completed the FIT in the third year of data collection (i.e., the final assessment point used in the current study [T3]; $n = 108$) was conducted. Parents who completed the FIT at T3 reported completing more years of education than those who did not complete the FIT, $t(214) = -2.48$, $p < 0.05$. No significant group differences were found on any other variables included in the present analyses, including intervention condition or in demographic variables (i.e., child gender, child age, parent race/ethnicity).

Primary Analyses

We first evaluated a multilevel latent growth model including latent ineffective discipline intercept and slope factors estimated at both the parent–child dyad level and the housing site level. This model included four demographic covariates

Table 3.1 Descriptive statistics and correlations

Measure	T0 ineffective discipline ($n = 155$)	T1 ineffective discipline ($n = 136$)	T2 ineffective discipline ($n = 118$)	T3 ineffective discipline ($n = 108$)	BASC-2 child externalizing ($n = 215$)	BSI parental depression ($n = 215$)	PRQ parenting confidence ($n = 212$)	PRQ attachment ($n = 212$)
T0 ineffective discipline	–							
T1 ineffective discipline	0.32*	–						
T2 ineffective discipline	0.09	0.17	–					
T3 ineffective discipline	0.28*	0.17	0.26*	–				
BASC-2 child externalizing	0.32**	0.04	0.12	0.01	–			
BSI parental depression	−0.05	−0.22***	−0.06	−0.20***	0.14***	–		
PRQ parenting confidence	−0.20***	−0.02	−0.05	0.16	−0.47**	−0.32**	–	
PRQ attachment	−0.16***	−0.04	0.03	0.10	−0.35**	−0.15***	0.58**	-
Female gender	−0.09	−0.08	−0.15	0.06	−0.03	−0.03	−0.03	−0.02
Parent education (years)	−0.08	−0.09	−0.11	−0.28*	0.06	0.00	0.05	0.17***
Child age at T0	0.03	0.22***	0.01	0.13	−0.05	0.06	−0.01	0.03
European American ethnicity	0.11	0.00	−0.03	−0.21***	0.27**	0.05	−0.22*	−0.04
Mean	2.39	2.20	2.22	2.38	59.30	54.66	44.51	45.38
Standard deviation	0.73	0.56	0.53	0.47	12.44	9.61	10.90	10.40

Note. *T0* Time 0 (baseline), *T1* Time 1 (after 1 year of intervention), *T2* Time 2 (after 2 years of intervention), *T3* Time 3 (1-year follow-up post-intervention), *BASC-2* Behavior Assessment System for Children, Second Edition, *BSI* Brief Symptom Inventory, *PRQ* Parenting Relationship Questionnaire
*$p < 0.01$; **$p < 0.001$; ***$p < 0.05$

(i.e., parent race/ethnicity, parent education, child gender, child age) and four child/parent covariates (i.e., child behavior problems, parental depression, parenting self-efficacy, parent–child attachment). The within-level latent ineffective discipline slope was regressed onto each covariate. Each covariate was allowed to covary with the latent ineffective discipline intercept. The between-level slope was regressed onto intervention status. The main effects model including all covariates demonstrated an adequate fit for the data on some fit indices and a marginal fit on other indices, $\chi^2(51) = 71.27, p = 0.03$; CFI = 0.91; RMSEA = 0.042; SRMR = 0.077. Child behavior problems was the only significant predictor of the within-level latent ineffective discipline slope, $b = -0.003, p < 0.05$. Higher levels of externalizing behavior at baseline were associated with greater reductions in ineffective discipline over the 3 years of the study. Intervention condition was not a significant predictor of the between-level ineffective discipline slope.

We next estimated interaction models. Each interaction term between the child/parent variables and intervention condition was first entered individually to the main effects model. When added separately to the main effects model, two interaction terms, child behavior problems X intervention condition and parental depression X intervention condition were each significant predictors of the within-level latent slope within their respective models. These two interaction terms were retained for the final model. The interaction terms involving intervention condition and parenting self-efficacy and parent–child attachment did not explain significant variance in the slope. Because these variables did not contribute as main effect predictors or as interaction terms, they were dropped from the final model.

Figure 3.1 depicts the final interaction model. The model was an acceptable fit for the data, $\chi^2(58) = 51.78, p = 0.70$; CFI = 1.00; RMSEA = 0.00; SRMR = 0.085. In the within parent–child dyad model, child gender was reliably associated with the ineffective discipline intercept, cov $= -0.028, p < 0.05$. Parents of female children tended to have lower initial levels of ineffective discipline. The child behavior problems variable was also associated with the ineffective discipline intercept, cov $= 1.90, p < 0.001$. Parents of children with higher levels of externalizing behaviors tended to have higher initial levels of ineffective discipline. Also in the within model, parent minority status was a significant predictor of ineffective discipline slope, $b = -0.10, p < 0.05$. Caucasian parents tended to demonstrate greater reductions in ineffective discipline over the course of the study than parents of other racial/ethnic groups. Child behavior problems remained a significant predictor of ineffective discipline slope, $b = -0.006, p < 0.001$.

The model revealed a significant interaction term between baseline child behavior problems and intervention status in predicting ineffective discipline slope, $b = 0.005, p < 0.01$. Figure 3.2a illustrates this interaction. For parents in both the intervention and control groups, higher levels of initial baseline child externalizing behaviors were associated with greater improvements in discipline over the 3 years of the study (i.e., lower slopes). However, among parents of children with high levels of externalizing behavior, those parents in the intervention group showed greater reductions in ineffective discipline over the course of the study when compared to parents in the control group. Thus, when comparing outcomes

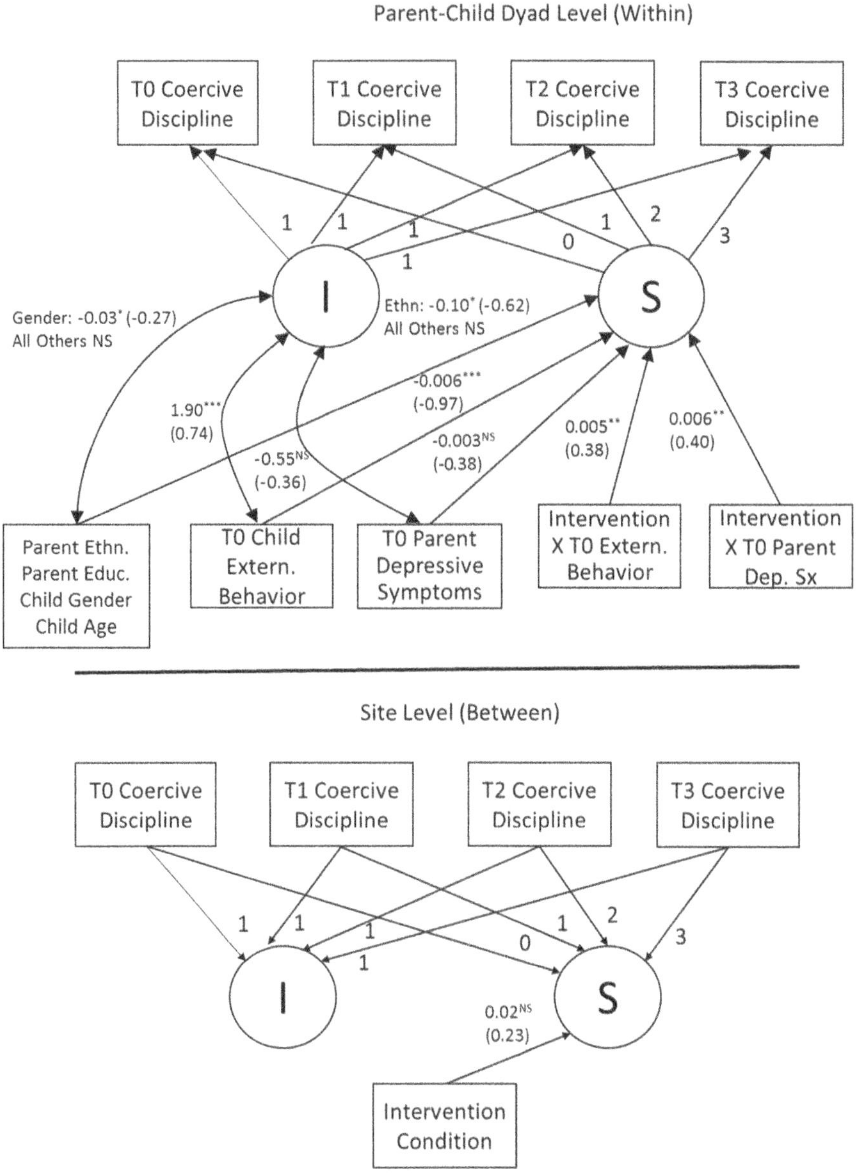

Fig. 3.1 Final multilevel latent growth model of observed ineffective discipline including maternal depression and child externalizing behavior covariates and interaction terms with intervention condition. *Note*. *I* intercept, *S* slope; Unstandardized factor loadings are depicted (with standardized parameters included in parentheses). *NS* non-significant. $*p < 0.05$; $**p < 0.01$; $***p < 0.001$. $n = 223$. Fit statistics: $\chi^2(58) = 51.78$, $p = 0.70$; CFI = 1.00; SRMR = 0.08

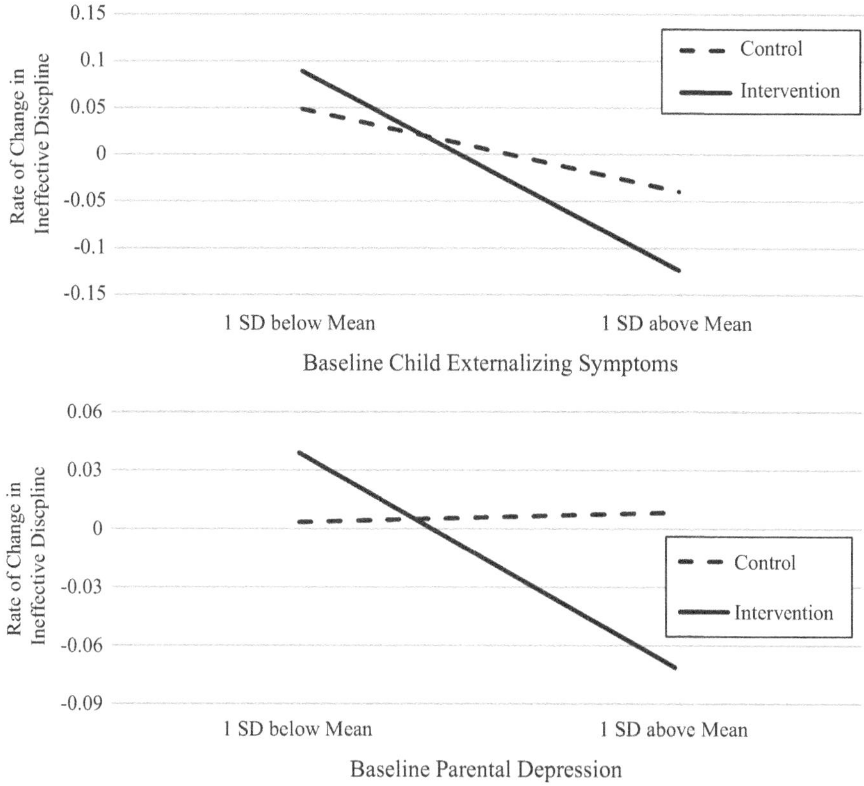

Fig. 3.2 (**a**) Interaction between intervention condition and baseline child externalizing symptoms in predicting rate of change in observed ineffective discipline. (**b**) Interaction between intervention condition and baseline parental depression in predicting rate of change in observed ineffective discipline

between conditions, parents of children with high levels of externalizing behavior demonstrated the most benefit in their discipline practices from participation in the intervention.

The model also revealed a significant interaction between intervention status and baseline parental depression in predicting ineffective discipline slope, $b = 0.006$, $p < 0.01$. The interaction is plotted in Fig. 3.2b. For parents in the intervention condition, higher levels of baseline depressive symptoms predicted greater improvements over the 3 years of the study in ineffective discipline than those parents reporting few depressive symptoms. For those parents in the control condition, level of depressive symptoms had little impact on their rate of change in ineffective discipline. When comparing outcomes (i.e., ineffective discipline slope) between intervention and control groups, those parents with high levels of depression exhibited the largest benefit in discipline practices from participation in the intervention.

Discussion

This study sought to identify child and parent characteristics predicting differential responses to a psychosocial preventive intervention among formerly homeless families in supportive housing. This was accomplished by testing moderation effects within the context of a randomized effectiveness trial. Observed ineffective discipline across four waves of assessment were examined using multilevel latent growth modeling to allow for analysis of data nested within parent–child dyads, families, and supportive housing sites. The findings were partially in support of the hypothesized moderators, indicating child behavior problems and parental depression each influenced the effect of the Early Risers intervention on change in observed parenting practices.

For both child behavior problems and parental depression, families experiencing the greatest level of initial distress fared the best in the intervention condition, observed in terms of steeper reductions in ineffective discipline practices compared to the control group. In fact, over the 3 years of the study, high distress families in the intervention condition showed greater improvements in observed parenting than any other group. These findings are not without precedent. Prior research has suggested families of children with more behavior problems (August et al., 2002; August et al., 2003) and those with a more depressed parent (Gardner et al., 2010) derive greater benefit from intervention participation in terms of improvements in child behavior. The current study extends these results by demonstrating these greater gains are also apparent in observed parenting practices. This is an exciting addition to the literature suggesting that psychosocial preventive interventions, such as Early Risers, are capable of serving at-risk families facing high levels of distress.

The potential moderating role of parenting self-efficacy and parent–child attachment was also examined in this study, but neither was supported. This finding is consistent with other studies which have not found support for parenting self-efficacy as a moderator of treatment outcome (McTaggart & Sanders, 2007; Spoth et al., 1995). Interestingly, research has suggested the influence of parenting self-efficacy on child outcomes is mediated by maternal depression (Weaver, Shaw, Dishion, & Wilson, 2008). When considered alongside extant intervention research (e.g., Gewirtz et al., 2015; McTaggart & Sanders, 2007), it seems parenting self-efficacy may exert an effect on parenting practices and child behavior through a complex causal chain operating over time, rather than acting in a moderating role. The lack of a significant result with regard to the moderating effect of parent–child attachment also adds to existing literature, which to date has largely focused on interventions targeting the early parent–child relationship and produced inconsistent results (e.g., Berlin et al., 2011; Feinberg & Kan, 2008). Study results suggest initial parent–child attachment does not predict differential responses to a psychosocial preventive intervention among formerly homeless families with school-age children.

Some additional findings also emerged. Child gender and baseline level of child behavior problems were each significantly associated with initial levels of ineffective discipline, such that parents of male children and parents of children with more externalizing behavior demonstrated greater ineffective discipline at the start of the study. Other research has shown a tendency for male children to receive harsher discipline than their female counterparts and has established a positive association between harsh discipline and child behavior problems (McKee et al., 2007). The current study extends these findings with a broader measure of ineffective discipline, beyond just harsh discipline, and among formerly homeless families in supportive housing.

The findings also highlight interesting main effects regarding change in ineffective discipline over time. Parents of children with more behavioral problems at baseline showed greater reductions in ineffective discipline over the course of the study, regardless of intervention condition. This is an encouraging finding suggesting homeless families experiencing an upheaval in child behavior problems tend to improve after entering supportive housing. This speaks to the capacity for resilience among homeless families (Cutuli & Herbers, 2014; Holtrop et al., 2015) as well as the potential effectiveness of supportive housing (i.e., housing plus case management services) in bolstering family functioning. Future research should substantiate and explore this finding, examining the mechanisms of this improvement to ensure it represents more than just a regression to the mean phenomenon. A less encouraging finding was that Caucasian parents seem to have shown more improvement in ineffective discipline than parents of racial/ethnic minority status. It could be families of color were facing additional challenges to positive parenting, such as discrimination, not accounted for in this study. Research with African American mothers has shown that facing high levels of discrimination can exacerbate the negative impact stressor pileup has on maternal psychological functioning and parent–child relationships (Murry, Brown, Brody, Cutrona, & Simons, 2001). It is also possible bias was present within the observational coding, yet such a bias would have been expected to lead to a difference in the ineffective discipline intercept as well.

The findings should be considered in light of study limitations. The families in this sample were overwhelmingly headed by a single, female parent. While this aligns with the typical demographic profile of homeless families in the USA (U.S. Department of Housing and Urban Development, 2012), care should be taken in extending study findings to other family types. While the use of observational methods to assess parenting practices represented a notable study strength, all hypothesized moderators were assessed through parent report. Relying only on parent report could introduce reporter biases to the measurement of these constructs. This study also encountered considerable attrition over the four waves of data collection, which was not unexpected given the transitional context of homeless families. The use of a cluster-randomized trial design is a limitation with respect to power. The use of this design, while necessary due to logistical considerations, limits the ability to successfully detect intervention effects.

Implications for Practice and Policy

The results of this research suggest important implications for intervention delivery among homeless populations meant to optimize impact on parenting practices. The focal intervention in this study demonstrated greater effectiveness for parents of children with more severe behavior problems and depressed parents. Although some practitioners may be reluctant to refer more highly distressed families to services, not wanting to unduly burden the family or intervention staff, the results of our study suggest these more highly distressed families actually stand to gain the most from intervention participation. Parents of children with more behavioral problems and depressed parents may be the most likely to benefit from comprehensive prevention programming and should be most actively recruited and engaged within these types of services. Yet the process of identifying these families may be complex. Families likely experience disruptions in functioning as they move into a shelter setting, and it is important to identify those truly in need of services without interfering with the adaptive capacity of family systems (Cutuli & Herbers, 2014). As our findings attest, families of children with more severe behavior problems tended to improve in discipline practices over time, regardless of intervention condition. This speaks to the need for sensitive assessment processes that can identify certain characteristics (i.e., child behavior problems, parental depression) that suggest families stand to gain meaningful benefits from intervention participation, as opposed to a one-size-fits-all approach that assumes all homeless families are in need of intensive treatment.

Study results may also help to inform policy. We echo the call of other scholars to implement and evaluate evidence-based programming with families exposed to homelessness (Haskett et al., 2016; Herbers & Cutuli, 2014). Our study findings can further guide these efforts, by underscoring the need to examine subgroups of responders to better understand for whom programming is most effective. In the case of this Early Risers effectiveness trial, despite other positive findings, no main effects of the intervention on observed parenting outcomes were found at 2 years post-baseline, using intent-to-treat analyses (Gewirtz et al., 2015). However, the current study identified parent and child characteristics that differentially predicted response to treatment after 3 years. When developing policy, it is important to recognize the effectiveness of these types of comprehensive interventions may not always be evident when evaluating the response of participants using intent-to-treat analyses, and that further investigation into the types of families best served by an intervention may be critical for meeting the needs of this heterogeneous population. Overall, the results of our study are encouraging. They indicate homeless families seemingly most at risk—those with children with more severe behavior and those with depressed parents—may be the most responsive efforts to improve parenting practices. This suggests the importance of allocating financial support and other resources toward efforts to reach out to those high-risk families with effective programming.

By investing in evidence-based interventions capable of promoting positive parenting among homeless families, we can help to stave off the negative repercussions of exposure to homelessness and support the mental health and developmental needs of homeless children.

References

Anderson, D. G., & Rayens, M. K. (2004). Factors influencing homelessness in women. *Public Health Nursing, 21*, 12–23. doi:10.1111/j.1525-1446.2004.21103.x.

Appleyard, K., & Osofsky, J. D. (2003). Parenting after trauma: Supporting parents and caregivers in the treatment of children impacted by violence. *Infant Mental Health Journal, 24*, 111–125. doi:10.1002/imhj.10050.

Arangua, L., Andersen, R., & Gelberg, L. (2005). The health circumstances of homeless women in the United States. *International Journal of Mental Health, 34*, 62–92. doi:10.1080/00207411.2005.11043398.

Assemany, A. E., & McIntosh, D. E. (2002). Negative treatment outcomes of behavioral parent training programs. *Psychology in the Schools, 39*, 209–219. doi:10.1002/pits.10032.

August, G. J., Realmuto, G. M., Hektner, J. M., & Bloomquist, M. L. (2001). An integrated components preventive intervention for aggressive elementary school children: The Early Risers program. *Journal of Consulting and Clinical Psychology, 69*, 614–626. doi: 10.1037/0022-006X.69.4.614.

August, G. J., Realmuto, G. M., Winters, K. C., & Hektner, J. M. (2001). Prevention of adolescent drug abuse: Targeting high-risk children with a multifaceted intervention model—The Early Risers "Skills for Success" Program. *Applied and Preventive Psychology, 10*, 135–154. doi:10.1017/S0962-1849(02)01005-3.

August, G. J., Hektner, J. M., Egan, E. A., Realmuto, G. M., & Bloomquist, M. L. (2002). The Early Risers longitudinal prevention trial: Examination of 3-year outcomes in aggressive children with intent-to-treat and as-intended analyses. *Psychology of Addictive Behaviors, 16*, S27–S39. doi:10.1037/0893-164X.16.4S.S27.

August, G. J., Lee, S. S., Bloomquist, M. L., Realmuto, G. M., & Hektner, J. M. (2003). Dissemination of an evidence-based prevention innovation for aggressive children living in culturally diverse, urban neighborhoods: The Early Risers effectiveness study. *Prevention Science, 4*, 271–286. doi:10.1023/A:1026072316380.

Baydar, N., Reid, M. J., & Webster-Stratton, C. (2003). The role of mental health factors and program engagement in the effectiveness of a preventive parenting program for Head Start mothers. *Child Development, 74*, 1433–1453. doi:10.1111/1467-8624.00616.

Berlin, L. J., Whiteside-Mansell, L., Roggman, L. A., Green, B. L., Robinson, J., & Spieker, S. (2011). Testing maternal depression and attachment style as moderators of Early Head Start's effects on parenting. *Attachment & Human Development, 13*, 49–67. doi:10.1080/14616734.2010.488122.

Chamberlain, P., Price, J., Leve, L. D., Laurent, H., Landsverk, J. A., & Reid, J. B. (2008). Prevention of behavior problems for children in foster care: Outcomes and mediation effects. *Prevention Science, 9*, 17–27. doi:10.1007/s11121-007-0080-7.

Cutuli, J. J., & Herbers, J. E. (2014). Promoting resilience for children who experience family homelessness: Opportunities to encourage developmental competence. *Cityscape: A Journal of Policy Development and Research, 16*, 113–139.

DeGarmo, D. S., Patterson, G. R., & Forgatch, M. S. (2004). How do outcomes in a specified parent training intervention maintain or wane over time? *Prevention Science, 5*, 73–89. doi:10.1023/B:PREV.0000023078.30191.e0.

Derogatis, L. R. (2000). *Brief Symptom Inventory (BSI) 18: Administration, scoring, and procedures manual*. Minneapolis, MN: NCS Pearson.

Duggan, A. K., Berlin, L. J., Cassidy, J., Burrell, L., & Tandon, S. D. (2009). Examining maternal depression and attachment insecurity as moderators of the impacts of home visiting for at-risk mothers and infants. *Journal of Consulting and Clinical Psychology, 77*, 788–799. doi:10.1037/a0015709.

Duncan, T. E., Duncan, S. C., Albert, A., Hops, H., Stoolmiller, M., & Muthen, B. (1997). Latent variable modeling of longitudinal and multilevel substance use data. *Multivariate Behavioral Research, 32*, 275–318. doi:10.1207/s15327906mbr3203_3.

Feinberg, M. E., & Kan, M. L. (2008). Establishing family foundations: Intervention effects on coparenting, parent/infant well-being, and parent-child relations. *Journal of Family Psychology, 22*, 253–263. doi:10.1037/0893-3200.22.2.253.

Forgatch, M. S., & DeGarmo, D. S. (1999). Parenting through change: An effective prevention program for single mothers. *Journal of Consulting and Clinical Psychology, 67*, 711–724. doi:10.1037/0022-006X.67.5.711.

Gardner, F., Burton, J., & Klimes, I. (2006). Randomised controlled trial of a parenting intervention in the voluntary sector for reducing child conduct problems: Outcomes and mechanisms of change. *Journal of Child Psychology and Psychiatry, 47*, 1123–1132. doi:10.1111/j.1469-7610.2006.01668.x.

Gardner, F., Hutchings, J., Bywater, T., & Whitaker, C. (2010). Who benefits and how does it work? Moderators and mediators of outcome in an effectiveness trial of a parenting intervention. *Journal of Clinical Child & Adolescent Psychology, 39*, 568–580. doi:10.1080/15374416.2010.486315.

Gewirtz, A. H. (2007). Promoting children's mental health in family supportive housing: A community-university partnership for formerly homeless children and families. *Journal of Primary Prevention, 28*, 359–374. doi:10.1007/s10935-007-0102-z.

Gewirtz, A., & Taylor, T. (2009). Participation of homeless and abused women in a parent training program. In M. F. Hindsworth, & T. B. Lang (Eds.), *Community participation and empowerment* (pp. 97–114). Hauppage, NY: Nova.

Gewirtz, A., Burkhart, K., Loehman, J., & Haukebo, B. (2014). Research on programs designed to support positive parenting. In M. E. Haskett, S. Perlman, & B. A. Cowan (Eds.), *Supporting families experiencing homelessness* (pp. 173–186). New York: Springer.

Gewirtz, A. H., DeGarmo, D. S., Lee, S., Morrell, N., & August, G. (2015). Two-year outcomes of the Early Risers prevention trial with formerly homeless families residing in supportive housing. *Journal of Family Psychology, 29*, 242–252. doi:10.1037/fam0000066.

Gewirtz, A. H., DeGarmo, D. S., Plowman, E. J., August, G., & Realmuto, G. (2009). Parenting, parental mental health, and child functioning in families residing in supportive housing. *American Journal of Orthopsychiatry, 79*, 336–347. doi:10.1037/a0016732.

Haskett, M. E., Loehman, J., & Burkhart, K. (2016). Parenting interventions in shelter settings: A qualitative systematic review of the literature. *Child and Family Social Work, 21*, 272–282. doi:10.1111/cfs.12147.

Hektner, J. M., August, G. J., Bloomquist, M. L., Lee, S., & Klimes-Dougan, B. (2014). A 10-year randomized controlled trial of the Early Risers conduct problems preventive intervention: Effects on externalizing and internalizing in late high school. *Journal of Consulting and Clinical Psychology, 82*, 355–360. doi:10.1037/a0035678.

Herbers, J. E., & Cutuli, J. J. (2014). Programs for homeless children and youth: A critical review of evidence. In M. E. Haskett, S. Perlman, & B. A. Cowan (Eds.), *Supporting families experiencing homelessness* (pp. 187–207). New York: Springer.

Holtrop, K., McNeil, S., & McWey, L. M. (2015). "It's a struggle but I can do it. I'm doing it for me and my kids": The psychosocial characteristics and life experiences of at-risk homeless parents in transitional housing. *Journal of Marital and Family Therapy, 41*, 177–191. doi:10.1111/jmft.12050.

van den Hoofdakker, B. J., Nauta, M. H., van der Veen-Mulders, L., Sytema, S., Emmelkamp, P. M. G., Minderaa, R. B., & Hoekstra, P. J. (2010). Behavioral parent training as an adjunct to routine care in children with attention-deficit/hyperactivity disorder: Moderators of treatment response. *Journal of Pediatric Psychology, 35*, 317–326. doi:10.1093/jpepsy/jsp060.

Hu, L. T., & Bentler, P. M. (1999). Cutoff criteria for fit indexes in covariance structure analysis: Conventional criteria versus new alternatives. *Structural Equation Modeling, 6*, 1–55. doi:10.1080/10705519909540118.

Kamphaus, R. W., & Reynolds, C. R. (2006). *Parenting Relationship Questionnaire manual*. Minneapolis, MN: NCS Pearson Inc..

Kim, M. M., Ford, J. D., Howard, D. L., & Bradford, D. W. (2010). Assessing trauma, substance abuse, and mental health in a sample of homeless men. *Health & Social Work, 35*, 39–48. doi:10.1093/hsw/35.1.39.

Kline, R. B. (2005). *Principles and practice of structural equation modeling* (2nd ed.,). New York: Guilford Press.

Kusché, C. A., & Greenberg, M. T. (1994). *The PATHS curriculum*. Seattle: Developmental Research Programs, Inc..

Lundahl, B., Risser, H. J., & Lovejoy, M. C. (2006). A meta-analysis of parent training: Moderators and follow-up effects. *Clinical Psychology Review, 26*, 86–104. doi:10.1016/j.cpr.2005.07.004.

Marra, J. V., McCarthy, E., Lin, H. J., Ford, J., Rodis, E., & Frisman, L. K. (2009). Effects of social support and conflict on parenting among homeless mothers. *American Journal of Orthopsychiatry, 79*, 348–356. doi:10.1037/a0017241.

McKee, L., Roland, E., Coffelt, N., Olson, A. L., Forehand, R., Massari, C., ... Zens, M. S. (2007). Harsh discipline and child problem behaviors: The roles of positive parenting and gender. *Journal of Family Violence, 22*, 187–196. doi:10.1007/s10896-007-90770-6.

McNeil Smith, S., Holtrop, K., & Reynolds, J. (2015). Do positive parenting practices moderate parental mental health and child behavior among homeless families? *Family Relations, 64*, 606–620. doi:10.1111/fare.12166.

McTaggart, P., & Sanders, M. R. (2007). Mediators and moderators of change in dysfunctional parenting in a school-based universal application of the Triple-P Positive Parenting Programme. *Journal of Children's Services, 2*, 4–17. doi:10.1108/17466660200700002.

Menting, A. T., Orobio de Castro, B., & Matthys, W. (2013). Effectiveness of the incredible years parent training to modify disruptive and prosocial child behavior: A meta-analytic review. *Clinical Psychology Review, 33*, 901–913. doi:10.1016/j.cpr.2013.07.006.

Murry, V. M., Brown, P. A., Brody, G. H., Cutrona, C. E., & Simons, R. L. (2001). Racial discrimination as a moderator of the links among stress, maternal psychological functioning, and family relationships. *Journal of Marriage and Family, 63*, 915–926. doi:10.1111/j.1741-3737.2001.00915.x.

Muthén, L. K., & Muthén, B. O. (2012). *Mplus user's guide* (Seventh ed.,). Los Angeles, CA: Muthén & Muthén.

Nowak, C., & Heinrichs, N. (2008). A comprehensive meta-analysis of Triple P-Positive Parenting Program using hierarchical linear modeling: Effectiveness and moderating variables. *Clinical Child and Family Psychology Review, 11*, 114–144. doi:10.1007/s10567-008-0033-0.

O'Connor, E., Rodriguez, E., Cappella, E., Morris, J., & McClowry, S. (2012). Child disruptive behavior and parenting efficacy: A comparison of the effects of two models of insights. *Journal of Community Psychology, 40*, 555–572. doi:10.1002/jcop.21482.

Perlman, S., Cowan, B., Gewirtz, A., Haskett, M., & Stokes, L. (2012). Promoting positive parenting in the context of homelessness. *American Journal of Orthopsychiatry, 82*, 402–412. doi:10.1111/j.1939-0025.2012.01158.x.

Piehler, T. F., Bloomquist, M. L., August, G. J., Gewirtz, A. H., Lee, S. S., & Lee, W. S. C. (2014). Executive functioning as a mediator of conduct problems prevention in children of formerly homeless families residing in temporary supportive housing: A parallel process latent growth modeling approach. *Journal of Abnormal Child Psychology, 42*, 681–692. doi: 10.1007/s10802-013-9816-y.

Piehler, T. F., Lee, S. S., Bloomquist, M. L., & August, G. J. (2014). Moderating effects of parental well-being on parenting efficacy outcomes by intervention delivery mode of the Early Risers Conduct Problems Prevention Program. *Journal of Primary Prevention*, *35*, 321–337. doi:10.1007/s10935-014-0358-z.

Prelow, H. M., Weaver, S. R., Swenson, R. R., & Bowman, M. A. (2005). A preliminary investigation of the validity and reliability of the Brief Symptom Inventory-18 in economically disadvantaged Latina American mothers. *Journal of Community Psychology*, *33*, 139–155. doi:10.1002/jcop.20041.

Rayburn, N. R., Wenzel, S. L., Elliott, M. N., Hambarsoomians, K., Marshall, G. N., & Tucker, J. S. (2005). Trauma, depression, coping, and mental health service seeking among impoverished women. *Journal of Consulting and Clinical Psychology*, *73*, 667–677. doi:10.1037/0022-006X.73.4.667.

Reyno, S. M., & McGrath, P. J. (2006). Predictors of parent training efficacy for child externalizing behavior problems–a meta-analytic review. *Journal of Child Psychology and Psychiatry*, *47*, 99–111. doi:10.1111/j.1469-7610.2005.01544.x.

Reynolds, C. R., & Kamphaus, R. W. (2004). *Behavior assessment system for children* (2nd ed.,). Circle Pines, MN: AGS.

Robinson, J. L., & Emde, R. N. (2004). Mental health moderators of Early Head Start on parenting and child development: Maternal depression and relationship attitudes. *Parenting: Science and Practice*, *4*, 73–97. doi:10.1207/s15327922par0401_4.

Spoth, R., Redmond, C., Haggerty, K., & Ward, T. (1995). A controlled parenting skills outcome study examining individual difference and attendance effects. *Journal of Marriage and the Family*, *57*, 449–464. doi:10.2307/353698.

Torquati, J. C. (2002). Personal and social resources as predictors of parenting in homeless families. *Journal of Family Issues*, *23*, 463–485. doi:10.1177/0192513X02023004001.

U.S. Department of Housing and Urban Development (2012). *The 2011 annual homeless assessment report to congress, revised*. Washington, DC: Author.

Weaver, C. M., Shaw, D. S., Dishion, T. J., & Wilson, M. N. (2008). Parenting self-efficacy and problem behavior in children at high risk for early conduct problems: The mediating role of maternal depression. *Infant Behavior and Development*, *31*, 594–605. doi:10.1016/j.infbeh.2008.07.006.

Zlotnick, C., Tam, T., & Bradley, K. (2007). Impact of adulthood trauma on homeless mothers. *Community Mental Health Journal*, *43*, 13–32. doi:10.1007/s10597-006-9070-7.

Chapter 4
Assessment of Families Experiencing Homelessness: Analysis of Current Practice

Carmela J. DeCandia, Ellen L. Bassuk, and Molly Richard

Introduction

Assessment lies at the core of our work with homeless families. To end homelessness, providers must understand families' needs, goals, and priorities. Without this information, developing a responsive service plan is impossible. To resolve a family's housing crisis and ensure outcomes that include residential stability, economic self-sufficiency, and child and family well-being, the work must begin with a well-crafted assessment.

Assessing family members is a relational activity between providers and clients (Rose, 2010); its purpose is to identify problems, needs, strengths, and resources and then determine a comprehensive and appropriate response (Department of Health and Social Security, 1981; Hoswarth, 2010). Assessment is not an easy task. Providers must understand the population being served and the context of their lives, and be able to develop trusting relationships while collecting sensitive information.

Despite insufficient funding, providers work hard to meet the needs of homeless families, most of whom have been repeatedly exposed to various traumatic stressors (Bassuk et al., 1996; Bassuk, Weinreb, Dawson, Perloff, & Buckner, 1997;

Author Note: The authors wish to acknowledge Homes For Families, Inc. in Boston, MA who focused attention on the need for comprehensive assessments of homeless families and sponsored a brief on the subject to inform policymakers and providers, and the Center for Social Innovation for supporting this project. Most importantly, we wish to thank all the providers across the country who graciously shared their intake and assessment protocols and answered our questions, so that we could gain a better understanding of current practice. We greatly appreciate their willingness to help inform and improve the assessment process for the benefit of homeless children and families.

C.J. DeCandia (✉)
Licensed Psychologist and Organizational Consultant, Newton, MA, USA
e-mail: cj@drdecandia.com

E.L. Bassuk • M. Richard
Center for Social Innovation, Needham Heights, MA, USA

M.E. Haskett (ed.), *Child and Family Well-Being and Homelessness*,
SpringerBriefs in Psychology, DOI 10.1007/978-3-319-50886-3_4

Hayes, Zonneville, & Bassuk, 2013). However, limited resources can impact the quality of the assessment. Without proper training it is often difficult for providers to ask the most relevant questions, rendering the assessment process less effective. For example, any assessment protocol must be informed by knowledge of the population so that the right questions are asked; furthermore, valid and reliable tools and instruments are needed to complement provider knowledge and to ensure that the most accurate information is gathered. The limited resources available to the homeless service workforce make conducting well-crafted, evidence-informed, and relationally based assessments challenging.

The complexity inherent in the lives of homeless families adds another layer to an already demanding job. Families experiencing homelessness are among the most marginalized in our society; the 2.5 million homeless children and their parents resemble a third world population within the United States (Bassuk, DeCandia, Beach, & Berman, 2014). These families not only struggle with severe poverty, un/underemployment, and lack of affordable housing, but also experience near universal exposure to interpersonal violence and trauma, and limited access to quality services (e.g., health, mental health, child care) (Bassuk et al., 2014; Hayes & DeCandia, 2012; Shipman & Taussig, 2009). As a result, many homeless mothers develop medical and mental health conditions, and their children often exhibit developmental delays and learning problems that go untreated for years (Bassuk et al., 2014). Such highly marginalized populations have complex, interrelated needs requiring assessments that incorporate an ecological perspective—simultaneously considering structural, familial, and individual needs of all family members.

All assessments are guided by questions; the clearer the question, the better the assessment. Historically, the homeless service system was developed to house adults who were living on the street or were chronically homeless. As homeless families began to emerge as a subpopulation, the same model was applied. The initial focus on situational and structural needs, namely housing and income, was essential but not sufficient. As the relationship among homelessness and residential instability, exposure to trauma, and the impact on children's development emerged (Guarino & Bassuk, 2010; Hayes et al., 2013; Herbers et al., 2011; Herbers & Cutuli, 2014; Samuels, Shinn, & Buckner, 2010), it has become clearer that the initial assessment paradigm must be expanded (DeCandia, 2015).

Research on the characteristics of homeless families (Bassuk et al., 1996, 1997; Browne, 1993; Browne & Bassuk, 1997; Rog & Buckner, 2007) and the impact of homelessness on children (Buckner, 2008; Buckner, Beardslee, & Bassuk, 2004; Hicks-Coolick, Burnside-Eaton, & Peters, 2003; Lindsey, 1998) indicates that families struggle with both structural (e.g., housing and income) needs and significant psychosocial issues. Consistent with previous research, a recent study of over 2000 homeless families including 5000 children (U.S. Department of Housing & Urban Development [HUD], 2015) confirmed the high rate (22%) of post-traumatic stress disorder (PTSD) and "serious psychological distress" (30%) among homeless parents (primarily mothers) (HUD, 2015). The study confirmed the consensus in the field (Bassuk, DeCandia, Tsertsvadze, & Richard, 2014; Bassuk & Geller, 2006) that long-term housing subsidies support family stability. However, the study failed to fully assess psychosocial and service needs such as maternal depression (Bassuk & Beardslee, 2014) and the mental health of the children (Bassuk, Richard, & Tsertsvadze, 2015). Without this knowledge, the study erroneously and dangerously concludes that most families do not need "specialized homeless-specific psychosocial services" (HUD, 2015, Executive Summary pp. xxx).

Based on the evidence, assessing homeless families involves asking four central questions: (1) What type and amount of structural supports are needed to resolve a family's homelessness? (2) What type and amount of services are needed to ensure that a family remains residentially stable and has improved well-being? (3) How are family members functioning? and (4) What are the children's needs?

Until recently, providers have been largely left on their own to answer these questions. Recognition of the need for a standardized assessment of homeless families has come from federal agencies. Most significantly, in 2013, HUD required that Continuums of Care (CoCs) develop and implement a centralized or "coordinated assessment" that includes a comprehensive, standardized assessment tool. Its purpose is to determine a client's eligibility for assistance, to quickly match the client to an appropriate housing option, and then to make appropriate referrals (HUD, 2013). To support the coordinated assessment process, newly available tools have emerged including the Service Prioritization Decision Assistance Tool for Families (F-SPDAT) and the Prescreen for Families (Organcode, 2013), and the Alliance Coordinated Assessment Tool Set (National Alliance to End Homelessness [NAEH], 2015). However, evidence for effectiveness of these tools does not yet exist.

As the number of families experiencing homelessness has steadily grown (Bassuk et al., 2014), so too has the need for evidence-based assessments. Currently, there are significant research gaps and variability in the practice of assessing homeless families. The purpose of this investigation was to begin to fill this knowledge gap by analyzing current assessment practices of providers serving homeless families across the United States. First, we broadly reviewed what is known about the risk factors for family homelessness. Next, we sampled various emergency shelters, transitional housing programs, and supportive housing programs, and collected the initial assessment/intake protocols from 55 geographically diverse programs. Based on knowledge of homeless families, we developed a protocol for determining the comprehensiveness and relevance of the assessments and reported the findings. We conclude with a discussion of how the study results can help close the research–practice gap and inform policy regarding assessments of homeless families.

Background

The profile of homeless families has remained consistent over the past two decades (Bassuk et al., 1996, 1997). Comprised of single mothers in their twenties with young children (HUD, 2009), they are extremely poor and struggle with limited education, jobs that do not pay a livable wage, unemployment, and difficulties accessing affordable child care (Wood & Paulsell, 2000). A disproportionate number of families are African-American and Latino and more than half of homeless children are under age 5 (HUD, 2009).

The research has also consistently reported on the high rates of interpersonal trauma and depression in the lives of homeless mothers (Bassuk et al., 1996; Weinreb, Buckner, Williams, & Nicholson, 2006; Hayes et al., 2013). Over 93% of homeless mothers have experienced trauma, primarily domestic violence and child abuse, in their lifetimes, and approximately one-third meet diagnostic criteria for post-traumatic stress disorder (PTSD) (Bassuk et al., 1996; Hayes et al., 2013). Depression often accompanies experiences of trauma for many women. Not surprisingly, approximately half of homeless mothers suffer from a clinical depression before and during their experience of homelessness (Bassuk & Beardslee, 2014); some estimates are as high as 85% (Weinreb et al., 2006).

Trauma and depression in mothers, when left untreated, adversely impact parenting. For example, among low-income single mothers receiving home visits, those with co-occurring post-traumatic stress disorder (PTSD) and depression demonstrate poorer maternal functioning, are less responsive to their children, and often are less sensitive to their children's needs (Ammerman, Putnam, Chard, Stevens, & Van Ginkel, 2012). Among homeless mothers, a history of trauma has been associated with negative parenting practices (Herbers, Cutuli, Monn, Narayan, & Masten, 2014; Perlman, Cowan, Gewirtz, Haskett, & Stokes, 2012). Additionally, mother's trauma symptom severity has been associated with residential instability, maternal depression, and poorer outcomes for children (Hayes et al., 2013).

Children who are homeless are a high-risk group. Research indicates that many struggle with developmental delays, learning, and behavioral health problems (Haskett, Armstrong, & Tisdale, 2015; Masten, Militois, Graham-Berman, Ramirez, & Neeman, 1993; Rog & Buckner, 2007). Ten to 26% of homeless preschoolers, and 24 to 40% of homeless school-age children, have mental health problems requiring clinical evaluation (Bassuk et al., 2015). Although many homeless children are resilient (Gewirtz, DeGarmo, Plowman, August, & Realmuto, 2009), especially those with strong parent–child bonds and effective parenting (Herbers, Cutuli, Lafavor, Vrieze, & Leibel, 2011; Herbers et al., 2014), most homeless children are not comprehensively assessed.

Standardized instruments to screen for parental depression, trauma, and developmental delays in children have typically not been used to assess homeless families. Instruments with strong psychometric properties can reduce provider variability and bias, improve the accuracy of information, and lead to better outcomes as compared to relying on provider judgment alone (Kelley & Bickman, 2009; Kelley, Bickman, & Norwood, 2010). As the science of child development has grown, the use of developmental screeners for very young children has received more attention from federal leaders. The Administration of Children and Families (ACF) created a screening tool compendium for shelter providers (Moodie et al., 2014), and now recommends that shelter providers incorporate "a system of regular developmental and behavioral screening into (the) community's coordinated assessment or program intake process" (U. S. Department of Health and Human services and the U.S. Department of Education, 2014).

Method

Sample

To determine the comprehensiveness of strategies used to assess family members experiencing homelessness, we collected 55 intake/assessment forms from a geographically diverse set of emergency shelters, transitional housing, and supportive housing programs serving these families. We developed a sample of convenience by initially using a mailing list of 2450 health and human service agencies compiled by a national nonprofit organization. With the mailing list organized by state, we selected four programs within each state that served families experiencing homelessness. For states with more than four eligible programs, we selected the first four in alphabetical order; for states with fewer than four eligible programs, we identified additional programs using the Homeless Shelter Directory (homelessshelterdirectory.org). Once we arrived at 200 geographically diverse programs, we then randomly selected 50% ($N = 100$) of programs using Microsoft Excel's random value generator. To be eligible for inclusion in this study, a program had to offer emergency shelter, transitional housing, or housing with or without services to homeless families. Homeless families were defined as a parent (s) with one or more accompanying children or a pregnant mother; programs serving only homeless individuals or unaccompanied homeless youth were excluded.

Of our randomly selected list of 100 programs, 28 did not meet these inclusion criteria and were thus replaced by another program from the same state from the initial database of 200, or, if no program from that state remained, we used the Homeless Shelter Directory (homelessshelterdirectory.org). Of those replaced, seven served unaccompanied homeless youth; three served individual adults; eight only provided services to homeless families (e.g., case management), but excluded housing. In addition, three programs had closed, five did not perform intake/assessments (intake was done at a centralized location), one was in the process of changing forms, and one performed assessments online.

We conducted outreach to our sample through e-mails and phone calls in which we described the goal of our study and requested blank intake/assessment forms. Of the final 100 eligible programs that were contacted, we obtained forms from 55, for a response rate of 55%.

For the majority of non-responding programs, no e-mail or phone response was received. Others declined without reason, due to lack of time, or concerns about confidentiality. While various organizations offered multiple programs to families (e.g., shelter and transitional housing) and used the same assessment forms, three organizations sent distinct forms for two or three different program types. We evaluated these intake forms independently.

The 55 program intake/assessment forms included in the sample were received from 30 states. The majority of organizations consisted of a single program ($n = 46$), and others were multiservice organizations with more than one program type ($n = 9$). Single program organizations included emergency shelters ($n = 32$), domestic violence shelter ($n = 1$), transitional housing programs ($n = 6$), and permanent housing programs ($n = 7$). Multiservice organizations included agencies with both an emergency shelter and transitional housing program ($n = 4$); agencies with both an emergency shelter and permanent housing program ($n = 2$); agencies with both a transitional housing and permanent housing program ($n = 2$); and agencies with an emergency shelter, transitional housing, and permanent housing program ($n = 1$).

Measurement for Evaluating the Intake/Assessment Forms

Based on a general literature review of family homelessness (for complete list of references used in this review, please contact the first author) and a targeted review of the assessment literature focused on homeless families (DeCandia, 2015), we developed a rating tool for assessing the intake forms that was divided into the following domains: (1) demographics, (2) immediate safety needs, (3) housing and homelessness, (4) self-sufficiency, (5) service use, (6) parent functioning (health, mental health, substance use, trauma, criminal justice involvement, social supports, parenting), (7) child developmental status, and (8) use of standardized screening instruments (child development, trauma, depression, parenting, social supports). Within each of these categories, we included specific items that were rated yes/no ("yes" denoted that the domain in question was included in the assessment tool, "no" denoted that it was absent). We then summarized our findings within each domain as strong (>50% yes), adequate (50% yes), and deficient (<50% yes), and then aggregated these into an overall rating. See Table 4.1 for examples of domains 4 and 7. Two clinicians (CDC, EB) knowledgeable about family homelessness independently reviewed 20% of the sample ($n = 10$). The percent agreement was 100%. The remaining 45 forms were reviewed by one clinician (CDC).

Results

No intake/assessments were rated as strong. Overall, when considering all domains together, four were rated as adequate (>50% or more than four domains rated adequate), and 51 as deficient (≤50% or four or more domains rated as deficient). With regard to the domains, the majority of the domains comprising the intakes

Table 4.1 Sample items of assessment protocol rating tool

Domain 4, self sufficiency		
1. Employment status and income	__Yes	__No
2. Benefits (e.g., TAFDC amount, food stamps, WIC)	__Yes	__No
3. Parent's highest level of education	__Yes	__No
4. Parent currently enrolled in school or vocational training	__Yes	__No
5. Parent's employment history (e.g., jobs held past year)	__Yes	__No
6. Parent's job skills (e.g., computer skill, retail, etc.)	__Yes	__No
7. Parent's preferences (e.g., get a job, return to school)	__Yes	__No
8. Transportation (e.g., has a car, driver's license, public transportation)	__Yes	__No
9. Child care needs	__Yes	__No
Sample items for domain 7, child developmental status		
1. Developmental status (e.g., good/normal, delayed)	__Yes	__No
2. Physical health status (e.g., poor, fair, good, or a medical diagnosis)	__Yes	__No
3. Mental/behavioral health status (e.g., diagnosis)	__Yes	__No
4. Learning needs (e.g., learning difficulties)	__Yes	__No

Table 4.2 Composite and domain ratings of assessment protocols

	Rating		
	Strong	Adequate	Deficient
Composite scores	0	7% ($n = 4$)	93% ($n = 51$)
Family demographics	0	42% ($n = 23$)	58% ($n = 32$)
Safety	0	20% ($n = 11$)	80% ($n = 44$)
Housing and homelessness	0	35% ($n = 19$)	65% ($n = 36$)
Self-sufficiency	0	35% ($n = 19$)	65% ($n = 36$)
Service use	0	27% ($n = 15$)	73% ($n = 40$)
Parent functioning	0	18% ($n = 10$)	82% ($n = 45$)
Child developmental status	0	18% ($n = 10$)	82% ($n = 45$)
Screening instruments	0	4% ($n = 2$)	96% ($n = 53$)

were rated as deficient. Approximately one-third of the categories of demographics, housing and homelessness, and self-sufficiency were rated as adequate. See Table 4.2 for the composite scores as well as the scores in each domain.

Discussion: Implications for Practice and Policy

To our knowledge, this is the first study to systematically evaluate the initial intake and assessment process of emergency shelters, transitional programs, and permanent supportive housing serving homeless families. Our findings highlight the variability in the assessment process across programs, the lack of comprehensiveness and standardization of the intake process, the inattention to children's needs, and limited questions about the functional status of the parents and their service needs. While housing and factors related to self-sufficiency are more thoroughly addressed, they are still not comprehensively evaluated. Overall, only 7% of the 55 protocols that we assessed were scored as adequate; all others were considered deficient.

A review of individual domains suggested three additional issues: (1) race was not always considered and primary language was often omitted; (2) immediate safety needs of all family members were poorly assessed; and (3) parents' preferences, wishes, and desires for themselves and their families were almost always overlooked. Assessments should be informed by the evidence (DeCandia, 2015). As African-American and Latino families are overrepresented in the homeless system (HUD, 2012) and domestic violence is common among homeless families (U.S. Conference of Mayors, 2011), these factors are especially important. In addition, best practice indicates that consumer choice should direct the course of services (Hopper, Bassuk, & Olivet, 2010), a key ingredient of family-centered, trauma-informed, culturally competent care of homeless families (DeCandia, 2015).

Several limitations should be considered when interpreting the results. We used a small sample of convenience with no comparison group, and the response rate was 55%. Although the selection of sites was randomized by state, it remains a sample of convenience and its generalizability is therefore limited. Furthermore, the assessment forms revealed considerable variability in how programs collect information. For many, the forms we gathered were the sole protocols used, while for others they represented the first phase of an evolving assessment over time. This study focused only on the initial protocols. It was not possible to determine how many programs had additional steps in their assessment process.

The emergence of a coordinated assessment process in the past 2 years further complicates this picture. Some programs incorporated the Homeless Management Information System [HMIS] into their initial protocols while others viewed HMIS as a data collection system with individuals not identified; these latter programs considered HMIS data collection as a separate activity. Despite these limitations, the results of our study indicate that assessments of homeless families are highly variable and largely deficient; they do not capture the full range of immediate and longer-term needs of the parents and children.

Practice Implications

Research has clearly demonstrated that ending family homelessness involves more than supplying a key to an apartment; attention must be paid to how well a parent and her children are functioning (Bassuk et al., 2014). To date, research indicates that current housing and service interventions result in limited positive outcomes for homeless families; the majority of families do not become residentially stable or self-sufficient, and their well-being is not substantially improved (Bassuk & Geller, 2006; Bassuk et al., 2014).

Our study findings suggest that a more comprehensive assessment will help to highlight issues that must be addressed in order to ensure residential stability and improve family well-being. In most studies of homeless families, parent's mental health and children's functioning are not evaluated (Bassuk et al., 2014). However, when these factors are investigated, elevated rates of maternal trauma and depression and child developmental delays are evident (Haskett et al., 2015; Hayes et al., 2013). The link between maternal depression and a range of adverse child outcomes is well established (Goodman, 2007; Goodman et al., 2011; National Research Council and Institute of Medicine (NRC & IOM), 2009a). Depression and traumatic stress interfere with a mother's capacity to maintain stable housing and parent effectively, contributing to decreased resilience in children (Gewirtz et al., 2009; Herbers et al., 2011, 2014; Knitzer, Theberge, & Johnson, 2008). A robust evidence base indicates that strategies focused on improving parenting capacities can mitigate some of these outcomes (NRC & IOM, 2009a, 2009b). Emerging evidence indicates parenting programs for homeless families can support family and child well-being (Gewirtz, 2007; Gewirtz & Taylor, 2009). Thus, to best serve homeless families, it is recommended that providers routinely inquire about these factors.

Assessing parent functioning, parenting capacity, and developmental status is critical to designing effective individualized service plans for homeless families. This requires that assessments expand beyond a narrow focus on housing supports and include an assessment of parent and child functioning. Specialization in practice is a popular trend; it makes targeting resources easier (Smyth, Goodman, & Glenn, 2006). However, assessments that narrow their focus to only one or two issues (e.g., housing and income) risk missing critical problems that require attention. Narrowly focused assessments can mask the complexity of the issues and oversimplify the solution. When this kind of model is applied to highly vulnerable, marginalized families with multiple needs (e.g., homeless families), it results in compromised quality of care, fragmented service systems, and ill-equipped providers (Smyth et al., 2006). This approach tends to define the problem narrowly in an attempt to align with the lack of resources. Instead, the problem should be redefined to align with people's needs; this requires a comprehensive framework for assessing homeless families—one that assesses both housing and service needs and is family-centered (DeCandia, 2015).

Policy Implications

To date, the prevailing paradigm underlying how assessments of homeless families are typically constructed has been based on two central tenets: (1) homelessness is primarily a housing issue, services are secondary and to avoid duplication should be accessed in the mainstream; and (2) homelessness and interventions to address it are currently focused on the adults, often excluding the needs of the children. Recent research has indicated that housing is essential for ending family homelessness but it is not sufficient for ensuring ongoing family stability, self-sufficiency, and well-being (Bassuk & Geller, 2006; Bassuk et al., 2014). Although experts agree that decent affordable housing generally acquired with subsidies are essential for ending homelessness among families (Bassuk et al., 2014; HUD, 2015), there remains a debate in the field about the role of services (Bassuk, Volk, & Olivet, 2010). This perspective seems to be reflected in the general deficiency of the assessment protocols that were evaluated in this study.

The second tenet is located within a larger sociopolitical context that has historically misunderstood the needs of children and the critical role played by their caregivers in their development (National Scientific Council on the Developing Child, 2015). A major shortcoming in the assessment protocols evaluated in this study was the lack of attention paid to the children and the need for family-oriented interventions that are two generational—addressing the needs of parents and their children, as well as the relationship between the two (Chase-Lansdale & Brooks-Gunn, 2014; Kids Count, 2014; Mosle & Patel, 2012; St. Pierre, Layzer, & Barnes, 1995). Despite evidence indicating the critical importance of the parent–child relationship to the children's well-being (Herbers et al., 2011; Masten & Coatsworth, 1998; Shonkoff, 2010), the assessment protocols we evaluated paid little attention to this relationship. In effect, children continue to be seen as *"along for the ride"* (Bassuk et al., 2010).

Fortunately, this context is beginning to change. Over the past 10 years, research on the developing brain, especially related to very young children (Center on the Developing Child at Harvard University, 2007, 2009, 2010, 2015; Shonkoff, 2010; Shonkoff et al., 2012), has begun to influence policy (Center on the Developing Child at Harvard University, 2015). Alongside this shift, policymakers are also beginning to recognize the impact of traumatic stress on human behavior leading to emerging adaptations of trauma-informed care in public health, human service, and educational systems (DeCandia, Guarino, & Clervil, 2014; DeCandia & Guarino, 2015; Substance Abuse and Mental Health Services Administration (SAMHSA), 2014). Buoyed by evidence on how adverse childhood experiences (ACE) impact adult outcomes (Felitti et al., 1998), ACE are also now being investigated for their effect on children's resilience (Bethell, Newacheck, Hawes, & Halfon, 2014). Thus, it is imperative that policymakers support the use of assessments that are trauma-informed.

Historically, family homelessness has not been a priority among policymakers (Bassuk et al., 2014). Funding for housing subsidies has fallen far below need (National Low Income Housing Coalition, 2013a, 2013b, 2013c), little monies have been available for research, and providers have been resource deprived (Mullen & Leginski, 2010). The result is a poorly developed evidence base supporting the effectiveness of various interventions, no evidence-based practices for the population (Bassuk et al., 2014), few tools for providers, and assessments that are not comprehensive or informed by evidence. In addition, due to a lack of resources, federal leaders tend to focus too narrowly and limit the scope of the problem to manage scarce resources. Homeless families have borne the brunt of this approach. Unless we remedy this situation, the future of many homeless families will remain compromised.

Conclusion

Current assessment practices of families experiencing homelessness are highly variable and often lack critical elements. Overall, housing and economic needs are better assessed than the need for psychosocial services, although not uniformly. Service needs tend to focus more on structural supports with little attention paid to parent's mental health, parenting, and children's needs. In addition, current assessment practice does not reflect the tenets of person-/family-centered, trauma-informed, or culturally competent care (DeCandia, 2015). Three decades of research on the characteristics of homeless families (Bassuk et al., 1996, 1997; Bassuk, DeCandia, Tsertsvadze and Richard 2014; Hayes et al., 2013; Weinreb et al., 2006) strongly support the need for family-oriented assessments that consider both the structural issues impinging on these families and their psychosocial needs—and that the assessments must be two generational (DeCandia, 2015). The homelessness field can benefit from the advice of Shonkoff and colleagues at the Center on the Developing Child (2015). They write: *"Advances in the science of human development can be mobilized to inform a new wave of strategies for building the capabilities that help both children and adults thrive in the face of economic and social disadvantage"* (p. 8). It is time that homeless families receive the same attention. We can begin at the beginning, with comprehensive assessments that systematically assess housing and service needs of parents and their children. For families and the field as a whole, this is long overdue.

References

Ammerman, R. T., Putnam, F. W., Chard, K. M., Stevens, J., & Van Ginkel, J. B. (2012). PTSD in depressed mothers in home visitation. *Psychological Trauma*, *4*(2), 1–19. doi:10.1037/a0023062.

Bassuk, E. L., & Beardslee, W. (2014). Depression in homeless mothers: Addressing an unrecognized public health issue. *American Journal of Orthopsychiatry*, *84*, 73–81. doi:10.1037/h0098949.

Bassuk, E. L., & Geller, S. (2006). The role of housing and services in ending family homelessness. *Housing Policy Debate*, *17*, 781–806. doi:10.1080/10511482.2006.9521590.

Bassuk, E. L., DeCandia, C. J., Beach, C. A., & Berman, F. (2014). *America's youngest outcasts: A report card on child homelessness*. Waltham, MA: The National Center on Family Homelessness at American Institutes for Research. Retrieved from www.homelesschildrenamerica.org

Bassuk, E. L., DeCandia, C. J., Tsertsvadze, A., & Richard, M. K. (2014). The effectiveness of housing interventions and housing and service interventions on ending family homelessness: A systematic review. *American Journal of Orthopsychiatry*, *84*, 457–474. doi:10.1037/ort0000020.

Bassuk, E. L., Richard, M., & Tsertsvadze, A. (2015). The prevalence of mental illness in homeless children: A systematic review and meta-analysis. *Journal of the American Academy of Child and Adolescent Psychiatry*, *54*, 86–96. doi:10.1016/j.jaac.2014.11.008.

Bassuk, E. L., Volk, K., & Olivet, J. (2010). A framework for developing supports and services for families experiencing homelessness. *Open Health Services and Policy Journal*, *3*, 34–40. doi:10.2174/1874924001003010034.

Bassuk, E. L., Weinreb, L. F., Dawson, R., Perloff, J. N., & Buckner, J. C. (1997). Determinants of behavior in homeless and low-income housed preschool children. *Pediatrics*, *100*, 92–100. doi:10.1542/peds.100.1.92.

Bassuk, E. L., Weinreb, L., John, C. B., Browne, A., Salomon, A., & Bassuk, S. S. (1996). The characteristics and needs of sheltered homeless and low-income housed mothers. *Journal of the American Medical Association*, *276*, 640–646. doi:10.1001/jama.1996.03540080062031.

Bethell, C. D., Newacheck, P., Hawes, E., & Halfon, N. (2014). Adverse childhood experiences: Assessing the impact on health and school engagement and the mitigating role of resilience. *Health Affairs*, *33*, 2106–2115. doi:10.1377/hlthaff.2014.0914.

Browne, A. (1993). Family violence and homelessness: The relevance of trauma histories in the lives of homeless women. Special Section: Homeless women: Economic and social issues. *American Journal of Orthopsychiatry*, *63*, 370–384. doi:10.1037/h0079444.

Browne, A., & Bassuk, S. S. (1997). Intimate violence in the lives of homeless and housed women: Prevalence and patterns in an ethnically diverse sample. *American Journal of Orthopsychiatry*, *67*, 261–278. doi:10.1037/h0080230.

Buckner, J. (2008). Understanding the impact of homelessness on children challenges and future research directions. *American Behavioral Scientist*, *51*, 721–736. doi:10.1177/0002764207311984.

Buckner, J. C., Beardslee, W. R., & Bassuk, E. L. (2004). Exposure to violence and low-income children's health: Direct, moderated, and mediated relations. *American Journal of Orthopsychiatry*, *74*, 413–423. doi:10.1037/0002-9432.74.4.413.

Center on the Developing Child at Harvard University. (2007). *The science of early childhood development*. National Scientific Council on the Developing Child; pp. 1–13. Retrieved from http://developingchild.harvard.edu/resources/reports_and_working_papers/science_of_early_childhood_development/

Center on the Developing Child at Harvard University. (2009). *Maternal depression can undermine the development of young children* (Working Paper No. 8). Cambridge, MA: Harvard University. Retrieved from http://www.developingchild.harvard.edu

Center on the Developing Child at Harvard University (2010). *The foundations of lifelong health are built in early childhood*. Cambridge, MA: Harvard University.

Center on the Developing Child at Harvard University (2015). *A decade of science informing policy: The story of the National Scientific Council on the Developing Child*. Cambridge, MA: Harvard University.

Chase-Lansdale, P. L., & Brooks-Gunn, J. (2014). Two-generation programs in the twenty-first century. *The Future of Children*, *24*(1), 13–39.

Kids Count (2014). *Creating opportunity for families: A two generation approach*. Annie E. Casey Foundation. Retrieved from http://www.aecf.org/m/resourcedoc/aecf-CreatingOpportunityforFamilies-2014.pdf

DeCandia, C. J. (2015). *Assessment of homeless families: A guide for practitioners and policy makers*. Boston, MA: Homes for Families.

DeCandia, C. J., & Guarino, K. G. (2015). Trauma-informed care: An ecological response. *Journal of Child Care and Youth Work*, *25*, 7–32.

DeCandia, C. J., Guarino, K., & Clervil, R. (2014). *Trauma-informed care and trauma-specific services: A comprehensive approach to trauma intervention*. Waltham, MA: American Institutes for Research.

Department of Health & Social Security. (1981). Observation and assessment. Report of a working party. London: Author.

Felitti, V. J., Anda, R. F., Nordenberg, D., Wiliamson, D. F., Spitz, A. M., Edwards, V., ... Marks, J. S. (1998). Relationship of childhood abuse and household dysfunction to many of the leading causes of deaths in adults: The Adverse Childhood Experiences (ACE) Study. *American Journal of Preventive Medicine*, *14*(4), 245–258. doi:10.1016/S0749-3797(98)00017-8.

Gewirtz, A., & Taylor, T. (2009). Participation of homeless and abused women in a parent training program: Science and practice converge in a battered women's shelter. In M. F. Hindsworth, &

T. B. Lang (Eds.), *Community Participation and Empowerment* (pp. 97–114). New York: Nova Science.
Gewirtz, A. H. (2007). Promoting children's mental health in family supportive housing: A community-university partnership for formerly homeless children and families. *Journal of Primary Prevention, 28*, 359–374. doi:10.1007/s10935-007-0102-z.
Gewirtz, A. H., DeGarmo, D. S., Plowman, E. J., August, G. G., & Realmuto, G. (2009). Parenting, parental mental health, and child functioning in families residing in supportive housing. *American Journal of Orthopsychiatry, 79*, 336–347. doi:10.1037/a0016732.
Goodman, S. H. (2007). Depression in mothers. In S. Nolen-Hoeksema, T. D. Cannon, & T. Widiger (Eds.), *Annual review of clinical psychology* (vol. 3, pp. 107–135). Palo Alto: Annual Reviews.
Goodman, S. H., Rouse, M. H., Connell, A. M., Broth, M. R., Hall, C. M., & Heyward, D. (2011). Maternal depression and child psychopathology: A meta-analytic review. *Clinical Child and Family Psychology Review, 14*, 1–27. doi:10.1007/s10567-010-0080-1.
Guarino, K., & Bassuk, E. (2010). Working with families experiencing homelessness: Understanding trauma and its impact. *Zero to Three, 30*(3), 11–20.
Haskett, M. E., Armstrong, J., & Tisdale, J. (2015). Developmental status and social-emotional functioning of young children experiencing homelessness. *Early Childhood Education Journal, 44*, 119–125. doi:10.1007/s10643-015-0691-8.
Hayes, M., & DeCandia, C. J. (2012). *The SHIFT Study: A cost analysis of housing and services for families*. Needham, MA: National Center on Family Homelessness.
Hayes, M., Zonneville, M., & Bassuk, E. (2013). *The SHIFT Study final report: Service and housing interventions for families in transition*. Newton, MA: The National Center on Family Homelessness.
Herbers, J. E., & Cutuli, J. J. (2014). Programs for homeless children and youth: A critical review of evidence. In M. E. Haskett, S. Perlman, & B. A. Cowan (Eds.), *Supporting families experiencing homelessness: Current practices and future directions* (pp. 187–207). New York: Springer.
Herbers, J. E., Cutuli, J. J., Lafavor, T. L., Vrieze, D., & Leibel, C. (2011). Direct and indirect effects of parenting on the academic functioning of young homeless children. *Early Education and Development, 22*, 77–104. doi:10.1080/10409280903507261.
Herbers, J. E., Cutuli, J. J., Monn, A. R., Narayan, A. J., & Masten, A. S. (2014). Trauma, adversity, and parent-child relationships among young children experiencing homelessness. *Journal of Abnormal Child Psychology, 42*, 1167–1174. doi:10.1007/s10802-014-9868-7.
Hicks-Coolick, A. H., Burnside-Eaton, P., & Peters, A. (2003). Homeless children: Needs & services. *Child & Youth Care Forum, 32*, 197–210. doi:10.1023/A:1024112015196.
Hopper, E. K., Bassuk, E. L., & Olivet, J. (2010). Shelter from the storm: Trauma-informed care in homeless service settings. *The Open Health Services and Policy Journal, 3*, 80–100. doi:10.2174/1874924001003010080.
Hoswarth, J. (2010). *The child's world: The comprehensive guide to assessing children in need*. Philadelphia: Jessica Kingsley Publishers.
Kelley, S. D., & Bickman, L. (2009). Beyond outcomes monitoring: Measurement Feedback Systems (MFS) in child and adolescent clinical practice. *Current Opinion in Psychiatry, 22*, 363–368 s 2001. doi:10.1176/appi.ps.52.2.179.
Kelley, S. D., Bickman, L., & Norwood, E. (2010). Evidence-based treatments and common factors in youth psychotherapy. In B. L. Duncan, S. D. Miller, B. E. Wampold, & M. A. Hubble (Eds.), *The heart and soul of change: What works in therapy* (2nd ed., pp. 325–355). Washington, DC: American Psychological Association.
Knitzer, J., Theberge, S., & Johnson, K. (2008). *Reducing maternal depression and its impact on young children: Toward a responsive early childhood policy framework*. New York, NY: National Center for Children in Poverty.
Lindsey, E. W. (1998). The impact of homelessness and shelter life on family relationships. *Family Relations, 47*, 243–252. doi:10.2307/584973.

Masten, A. S., & Coatsworth, J. D. (1998). The development of competence in favorable and unfavorable environments: Lessons from successful children. *American Psychologist, 53*, 205–220. doi:10.1037/0003-066X.53.2.205.
Masten, A. S., Militois, D., Graham-Berman, S. A., Ramirez, M., & Neeman, J. (1993). Children in homeless families: Risks to mental health and development. *Journal of Consulting and Clinical Psychology, 61*, 335–343. doi:10.1037/0022-006X.61.2.335.
Moodie, S., Daneri, P., Goldhagen, S., Halle, T., Green, K., & LaMonte, L. (2014). *Early childhood developmental screening: A compendium of measures for children ages birth to five (OPRE Report 201411)*. Washington, DC: Office of Planning, Research and Evaluation, Administration for Children and Families, U.S. Department of Health and Human Services.
Mosle, A., & Patel, N. (2012, January). *Two generations, one future: Moving parents and children beyond poverty together*. Washington, DC: The Aspen Institute. Retrieved from http://www.aspeninstitute.org/sites/default/files/content/docs/ascend/Ascend-Report-022012.pdf
Mullen, J., & Leginski, W. (2010). Building the capacity of the homeless service workforce. *The Open Health Services and Policy Journal, 3*, 101–110.
National Alliance to End Homelessness [NAEH] (2015). *Assessment tools for allocating homelessness assistance: state of the evidence, Prepared for the U.S. Department of Housing and Urban Development [HUD], Office of Policy Development and Research*. D.C.: Washington.
National Low Income Housing Coalition (NLIHC) (2013a). *Housing spotlight: America's affordable housing shortage, and how to end it*. Washington, DC: Author.
National Low Income Housing Coalition (NLIHC). (2013b). *Out of reach 2013*. Washington, DC: Author. Retrieved from http://nlihc.org/oor/2013
National Low Income Housing Coalition (NLIHC). (2013c). *Advocates guide*. Washington, DC: Author. Retrieved from http://nlihc.org/sites/default/files/2014-Advocates-Guide.pdf
National Research Council and Institute of Medicine (NRC & IOM) (2009a). Depression in parents, parenting, and children: Opportunities to improve identification, treatment, and prevention. In M. J. England, & L. J. Sim (Eds.), *Committee on depression, parenting practices, and the healthy development of children*. Washington, DC: The National Academies Press.
National Research Council and Institutes of Medicine (NRC & IOM) (2009b). Preventing mental, emotional, and behavioral disorders among young people: Progress and possibilities. In M. E. O'Connell, T. Boat, & K. E. Warner (Eds.), *Committee on Prevention of Mental Disorders and Substance Abuse Among Children, Youth, and Young Adults: Research Advances and Promising Interventions*. Washington, DC: The National Academies Press.
National Scientific Council on the Developing Child. (2015). *Supportive relationships and active skill-building strengthen the foundations of resilience*. Working paper 13. Retrieved from http://www.developingchild.harvard.edu
OrganCode. (2013). Service Prioritization Decision Assistance Tool for Families (F-SPDAT). Organcode Consulting. Retrieved from: http://wnyhomeless.org/wp-content/uploads/VI-SPDAT-F.pdf
Perlman, S., Cowan, B., Gewirtz, A., Haskett, M. E., & Stokes, L. (2012). Promoting positive parenting in the context of homelessness. *American Journal of Orthopsychiatry, 82*, 402–412. doi:10.1111/j.1939-0025.2012.01158.x.
Rog, D. J., & Buckner, J. C. (2007). Homeless families and children. In D. Dennis, G. Locke, & J. Khadduri (Eds.), *Toward understanding homelessness: The 2007 National Symposium on Homelessness Research (Section 5.1)*. Cambridge, MA: Abt Associates.
Rose, W. (2010). The assessment framework. In J. Horwarth (Ed.), *The child's world: The comprehensive guide to assessing children in need*. Philadelphia: Jessica Kingsley Publishers.
Samuels, J., Shinn, M., & Buckner, J. C. (2010). *Homeless children: Update on research, policy, programs, and opportunities*. Washington, DC: Office of the Assistant Secretary for Planning and Evaluation, U.S. Department of Health and Human Services.
Shipman, K., & Taussig, H. (2009). Mental health treatment of child maltreatment and neglect. *Pediatric Clinics of North America, 56*, 417–428. doi:10.1016/j.pcl.2009.02.002.

Shonkoff, J. P. (2010). Building a new biodevelopmental framework to guide future early childhood policy. *Child Development, 81*, 357–367. doi:10.1111/j.1467-8624.2009.01399.x.
Shonkoff, J. P., Garner, A. S., Siegel, B. S., Dobbins, M. I., Earls, M. F., McGuinn, L., . . . Wood, D. L. (2012). The lifelong effects of early childhood adversity and toxic stress. *Pediatrics, 129* (1), e232–e246. doi:10.1542/peds.2011-2663.
Smyth, K. F., Goodman, L. A., & Glenn, C. (2006). The full-frame approach: A new response to marginalized women left behind by specialized services. *American Journal of Orthopsychiatry, 76*, 489–502. doi:10.1037/0002-9432.76.4.489.
St. Pierre, R. G., Layzer, J. I., & Barnes, H. V. (1995). Two-generation programs: Design, cost, and short-term effectiveness. *The Future of the Children, 5*(3), 76–93. doi:10.2307/1602368.
Substance Abuse and Mental Health Services Administration (SAMHSA) (2014). *Trauma-informed care in behavioral health services: A treatment protocol (TIP) Series 57, HHS Publication No. (SMA) 14–4816*. MD: Rockville.
U.S. Conference of Mayors (2011). *A status report on hunger and homelessness in America's cities*. Washington, DC: Author.
U.S. Department of Health and Human services and the U.S. Department of Education (2014). *Birth to five: Watch me thrive! A housing and shelter provider's guide to developmental and behavioral screening*. Washington, DC: Author.
U.S. Department of Housing & Urban Development [HUD] (2015). *Family options study: Short-term impacts of housing and services interventions for homeless families*. Washington, DC: Office of Policy Development and Research.
U.S. Department of Housing and Community Development. (2013). *CoC's coordinated assessment system Prezi*. Washington, DC: Author. Retrieved from https://www.hudexchange.info/resources/documents/CoCs-Coordinated-Assessment-System-Prezi-Slides.pdf
U.S. Department of Housing and Urban Development (HUD). (2012). *The 2012 annual homeless assessment report to congress: Volume 2—estimates of homelessness in the U.S.* Washington, DC: Author. Retrieved from https://www.hudexchange.info/resource/3297/2012-ahar-volume-2-estimates-of-homelessness-in-the-us/
U.S. Department of Housing and Urban Development [HUD] (2009). *The 2008 annual homeless assessment report to congress*. Washington, DC: Author.
Weinreb, L. F., Buckner, J. C., Williams, V., & Nicholson, J. (2006). A comparison of the health and mental health status of homeless mothers in Worcester, Massachusetts: 1993 and 2003. *American Journal of Public Health, 96*, 1444–1448. doi:10.2105/AJPH.2005.069310.
Wood, R. G., & Paulsell, D. (2000). *Employment retention for TANF recipients: Lessons from GAPS. Issue Brief, No. 1*. Princeton, NJ: Mathematica Policy Research. Retrieved from http://www.mathematica-mpr.com/PDFs/WTWIsBr1GAPS.pdf

Chapter 5
Access to Early Childhood Services for Young Children Experiencing Homelessness

Staci M. Perlman, Sara H. Shaw, Charles H. Kieffer, Grace-Ann C. Whitney, and Carie Bires

Introduction

Developmental science underscores the importance of the first years of life. During these years, young children develop the foundational cognitive, social–emotional, and gross/fine motor competencies that they will need to successfully negotiate developmental challenges across the life span (National Research Council and Institute of Medicine, 2000). These early years are also marked by increased vulnerability to traumatic events, including homelessness. Recent national estimates indicate that over 350,000 children and youth were served by emergency and transitional housing providers in 2012, and nearly 60% of these children were age five or younger (U.S. Department of Housing and Urban Development, 2013a). Furthermore, children are at greatest risk of entering the shelter system during the first year of life (Perlman & Fantuzzo, 2010).

Author Note: Data referenced in this chapter are based on two separate studies conducted by: (a) the National Association for the Education of Homeless Children and Youth and (b) The Cloudburst Group, under a contract with the U.S. Department of Housing and Urban Development (HUD) Office of Policy Development and Research (Grant#H-21616RG).

S.M. Perlman • S.H. Shaw (✉)
Department of Human Development and Family Studies,
University of Delaware, Newark, DE, USA
e-mail: shshaw@udel.edu

C.H. Kieffer
The Cloudburst Group, Landover, MD, USA

G.-A.C. Whitney
Connecticut Head Start Collaboration Office, Hartford, CT, USA

C. Bires
Ounce of Prevention, Chicago, IL, USA

M.E. Haskett (ed.), *Child and Family Well-Being and Homelessness*,
SpringerBriefs in Psychology, DOI 10.1007/978-3-319-50886-3_5

Research indicates that children born into homelessness are at risk for a number of adverse perinatal outcomes. Children are more likely to be born prematurely and at very low birth weight (Fantuzzo, LeBoeuf, Brumley, & Perlman, 2013; Little et al., 2005; Merrill, Richards, & Sloane, 2011; Richards, Merrill, & Baksh, 2011). Additionally, children born into homelessness are at increased risk for a stay in Neonatal Intensive Care Units (Richards et al., 2011). Furthermore, they are less likely to have well-baby visits and to be breastfed by their mothers (Little et al., 2005; Richards et al., 2011). These experiences have important implications for future development and may ultimately hinder healthy development.

Very young children are disproportionately more likely to spend some of the most developmentally important years of their lives without stable housing. Research demonstrates that the timing of homelessness during critical periods of development is important. To illustrate, in a study of over 10,000 third graders, children who experienced their first episode of homelessness during toddlerhood had a 60% increase in the odds of not meeting proficiency standards in math compared to children with homelessness experiences later in life (Fantuzzo et al., 2013). Experiencing homelessness in the first years of life also has been linked to poor health outcomes and developmental delay (Fantuzzo et al., 2013; Haber & Toro, 2004). Moreover, for school-aged children, experiences of homelessness have been associated with increased school problems, including poor academic achievement and high rates of behavior problems (Gewirtz, Hart-Shegos, & Medhanie, 2008; Perlman & Fantuzzo, 2010).

Prior research demonstrates that engagement in high-quality early childhood services can serve as a protective factor against these early risks (Puma et al., 2010). However, little is known about what factors facilitate/impede access to these services for young children experiencing homelessness. In that context, these two companion studies were designed to address several overlapping research questions: (1) Are providers and parents aware of early education services for young children experiencing homelessness and do parents receive support to access these services? (2) What factors impede access to early childhood services among young children experiencing homelessness? (3) What factors facilitate access to early childhood services? (4) In what ways does cross-systems collaboration facilitate homeless family participation in early childhood services? (5) What can be identified as promising practices among communities for facilitating access to early childhood services for families experiencing homelessness?

This chapter is based on data generated through an integrated mixed methods transformative design which included collecting and analyzing two independent strands of qualitative and quantitative data, and then seeking convergence, or relationships, between the two data sets (Creswell & Plano Clark, 2011). The purpose of a transformative design is to conduct research related to issues of social justice in order to enact change (Creswell & Plano Clark, 2011). The purpose of this merged analysis between the NAEHCY survey of homeless services and early childhood providers and The Cloudburst Group's (Cloudburst) HUD-funded qualitative study of homeless parents was to develop an understanding of key barriers and facilitators to accessing early childhood services (including child care,

Head Start, pre-K, and early intervention) for infants, toddlers, and preschoolers experiencing homelessness. The studies addressed these issues from the perspectives of (a) parents experiencing homelessness and (b) community-based services providers who were engaged with this population. In this design, both qualitative and quantitative data are analyzed concurrently and also independently. Select findings from each study have been reported previously (Perlman, 2014; Taylor, Gibson, & Hurd, 2015) but the data sets have not been explored through an integrated mixed methods transformative design.

Method

Participants and Procedures

NAEHCY is an organization originally established to support state and local school district liaisons under the McKinney–Vento Act (42 USC 11431 et seq) that has since grown to include among its membership personnel in Head Start programs, other early care and education programs, homelessness and housing services, and those in related roles within education and social services. In response to growing attention regarding the early education of young children experiencing homelessness, NAEHCY initiated a national survey designed to understand the challenges providers faced in accessing services for young children and to document promising practices those providers were implementing to address the challenges.

The survey was disseminated using Survey Monkey technology and the cumulative national listservs for NAEHCY and other national organizations. It was circulated several times over approximately 4 months between April and August 2013. The survey was completed by a convenience sample; unfortunately, it is not possible to estimate a response rate because the total number of people who were sent and received the e-mail invitation to complete the survey is not known. Responses were received from 970 providers who were asked to identify themselves by their role as a provider of services to children experiencing homelessness. Forty-six percent of the respondents were McKinney–Vento Homeless Education Liaisons, 27% were Early Head Start/Head Start professionals, 12% were child care providers, 11% were homeless housing providers, and the remaining respondents were from Local Education Agency preschool programs (LEAs).

At the same time as the NAEHCY survey was conducted, The Cloudburst Group—in a qualitative small research project sponsored by the Department of Housing and Urban Development (HUD) Office of Policy Development and Research (Grant #H-21616RG)—collected data on parental perspectives among recently homeless families about opportunities and barriers encountered regarding enrollment of their children into preschool, with a special focus on the relation between these decisions and processes and the families' experiences of homelessness.

The Cloudburst study drew on interviews with parents from 28 households in two varied geographic areas: Atlanta, Georgia and the Bridgeport/New Haven region of Connecticut. Interviews were conducted primarily between February and November of 2013. All study households were previously enrolled in the *Family Options Study*, a randomized control study funded and recently published by the Department of Housing and Urban Development (HUD). This larger study included 2307 homeless families across four housing/service interventions in 12 research sites across the United States (U.S. Department of Housing and Urban Development, 2013b). Cloudburst's qualitative study was designed as a smaller companion investigation tied to the broader national project, focused on increasing knowledge of how families who had experienced homelessness made decisions about preschool enrollment and participation. As national study enrollees were not immediately accessible to the research team due to privacy protections, the national study research team recruited voluntary participants. Only families with children under 6 years of age at the time of their enrollment in the *Family Options Study* were recruited to participate. Multiple invitations to participate in initial focus groups were mailed to several hundred eligible households in the two targeted geographic areas.

As a means of identifying basic demographic data descriptive of study participants, the research team relied on baseline data gathered by the national *Family Options Study* for each participant. Of the 28 heads of household/primary caretakers who participated in this study, 14 were interviewed in Connecticut and 14 were interviewed in Atlanta, Georgia. The average age of study participants was 31, ranging from 21 to 53 years old. Only one participant was married, 19 were never married, and seven were separated or divorced. Twenty-two participants were African-American, two were Caucasian, three were American Indian, and one was an unrecorded race. Fourteen participants had not completed high school, five had earned a high school or GED degree, eight had completed some college or earned an Associate's Degree or Technical Certificate, and one participant had a bachelor's degree.

Measures

Quantitative: Survey of early childhood and homeless services providers. In the quantitative study, conducted by Perlman (2014), providers of early education services for children aged birth to 5 years were targeted to complete a 53-item survey. Survey questions related to barriers to homeless families with young children accessing early childhood and homeless services; successful strategies for addressing those barriers; and collaboration among early childhood and homeless programs in addressing these issues. The survey asked providers to report their level of knowledge of various laws and early childhood programs, including the education provisions of the McKinney–Vento Homeless Assistance Act, preschool programs administered by local school districts, Early Head Start/Head Start, Early

Table 5.1 Provider ratings of familiarity with programs and laws

Program/law	Not at all familiar (%)	Somewhat familiar (%)	Very familiar (%)	*N*
Education provisions of McKinney–Vento Homeless Assistance Act	10.8	23.6	65.6	880
Preschool programs administered by a school district	6.9	31	62.1	870
Head Start/Early Head Start	5.6	34.5	59.9	877
Special Education Preschool (IDEA Part B)	10.3	37.2	52.5	871
Early Interventions (IDEA Part C)	10.4	41.6	48	864
Child care	8.7	43.5	47.9	865
Other early childhood programs	13.3	52.8	34	851

Intervention (Individuals with Disabilities Education Act Part C), Preschool Special Education (Individuals with Disabilities Education Act Part B), and other early childhood programs and services (see Table 5.1). Respondents rated their involvement with each program on a four-point scale. These ratings ranged from "no working relationship" to "collaboration" where respondents identified clear working relationships and shared resources with other partners (Perlman, 2014). The survey also explored providers' perspectives in assisting families experiencing homelessness and accessing related programs and services; identifying barriers to services enrollment; and examining strategies they had used to overcome those barriers. Other issues explored were provider involvement with various community programs and services; topics on which providers would like more information, and examples of effective programs and ideas for community-level strategies for better serving homeless families.

Qualitative: Interviews with parents experiencing homelessness. In the qualitative study conducted by Taylor et al. (2015), parents who had experienced homelessness were invited to take part in initial focus group dialogues and/or semi-structured individual interviews to prompt the reflections of participants on barriers to accessing early childhood services and experiences in identifying, pursuing, and participating in preschool settings for their 3–5-year-old children. Questions also explored the role that homeless program staff and early childhood service providers played in supporting families in pursuing preschool options. All interviews and focus groups were held two and three years after the participants' initial periods of homelessness. After the initial round of focus groups and introductory interviews was completed and preliminary data analysis had been conducted, the research team invited all participants from both sites to participate in one-on-one semi-structured follow-up interviews. Sixteen heads of households participated in these follow-up sessions. All interviews were audiotaped and transcribed for later coding.

Data Analytic Approach

Quantitative survey data were analyzed primarily using a series of frequency analyses to summarize the survey responses. To analyze the qualitative interview data, the Cloudburst team applied a modified grounded theory approach (Pope, Ziebland, & Mays, 2000). One of the coauthors of this chapter (CHK) was a Coprincipal Investigator for that study and contributed to that analysis as one of several coders. The research team carefully and independently read and reread transcripts to identify themes and subthemes emerging from the interviews, then aggregated and synthesized data from all transcribed files. After developing an analytical schema, the team completed detailed coding of transcripts from initial and follow-up interviews, extracting passages from transcripts illustrating emergent core themes. All data relevant to each theme and subtheme were identified and examined in comparison with all other related data reflected in other themes and subthemes. The coding process was iterative; that is, the research team reviewed and revised each categorization level multiple times, reflecting on nuances found in the data and then altering the articulation of themes as a consequence of this dynamic analysis. This protocol was used as a means to identify overarching categories and specific themes and subthemes that comprised the final coding structure for data analysis. This protocol also served as a mechanism for ensuring cross-rater neutrality and integrity.

For the present study, these two data sets were integrated in a mixed methods analysis of barriers and facilitators to accessing early childhood services for families experiencing homelessness. The integration of the data provides a richer and clearer understanding of the barriers to accessing early childhood services than would be possible using only one of the two data sources. Furthermore, the merging of these data sets provides a unique contribution to the understanding of access to early childhood services for children experiencing homelessness. Data were merged by comparing results from both studies and identifying themes in the findings. These data were integrated for the purpose of developing well-informed policy implications and recommendations to increase access to early childhood services (see Fig. 5.1).

Results

Systemic Barriers to Accessing Early Education Programs

Transportation. Both providers and parents suggested a number of barriers to accessing early education programming for children experiencing homelessness. Of all the barriers to accessing early education, the largest proportion of providers 29% (N=281) rated finding transportation as the strategy they were least successful in helping parents overcome (see Table 5.2). In fact, 27% (N= 262) of respondents

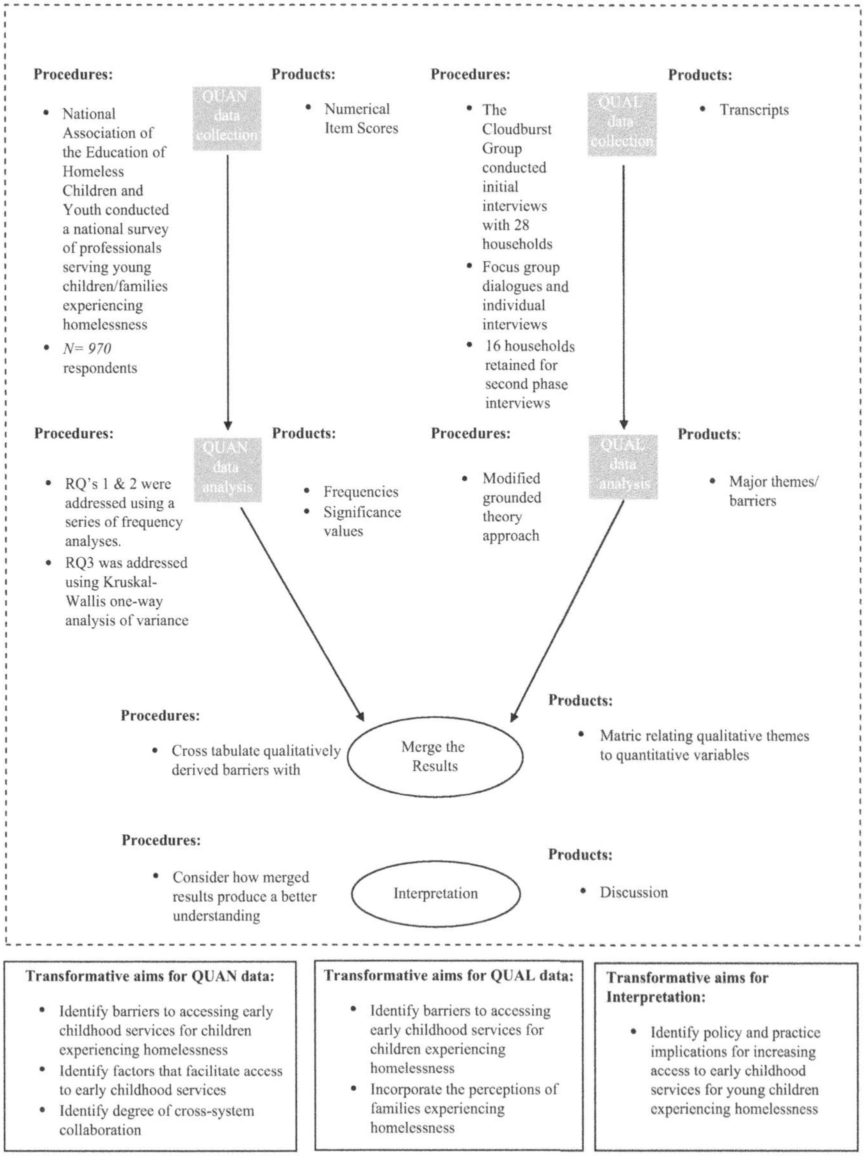

Fig. 5.1 A visualization of the mixed methods transformative design

endorsed this as a significant barrier. Several providers further qualified the transportation challenges facing parents, as follows: "*Preschool is not covered under transportation by the McKinney-Vento Act. If there is an older child in the district that they can bus, then the preschool child can bus. However, if it is only a preschool child they will not transport.*" Providers also indicated that this is an

Table 5.2 Provider ratings of success for strategies to connect families to EC programs

Strategy	Not successful (%)	Somewhat successful (%)	Very successful (%)	*N*
Help families complete paperwork	0.6	37.2	62.2	545
Help families obtain documentation and records	3.2	52.5	44.3	537
Develop relationships with EC programs	3.6	38.4	58	584
Develop relationships with homeless providers	4	39.2	56.8	553
Develop relationships with McKinney–Vento Liaisons	5.3	34.3	60.4	487
Conduct professional development training for EC programs	9.2	49.3	41.5	402
Conduct professional development training for housing providers	13.9	46.1	40	330
Dedicate staff person for early childhood issues	5.2	31.2	63.6	461
Have a key contact in various programs	5.1	39.8	55.1	548
Develop procedures to identify homeless children and families	6.4	40	53.6	500
Identify alternative transportation	29.1	41.4	29.5	478

even more pronounced burden in largely rural areas, where access to transportation is already limited.

Parents also self-reported multiple concerns regarding transportation barriers to access for early childhood education. Just over half of the parents in the Cloudburst study stated that they utilized public transportation or walked to the school. Other parents reported having their own means for transportation or relying on family and friends. Notably, only one parent received transportation services from the school itself. Further concerns with transportation were reflected in parents' desire to be closer to their child. This is reflected in a comment from a mother discussing concerns about her son's preschool location. *"So, you can't pay for transportation and you need somewhere you can walk to. These are things you gotta think (about). I gotta get my son somewhere if he gets hurt, I can get up there" (Madison, age 41).*

Finances. Another important consideration for parents was cost. *"I...wanted Head Start because in order to get...a child care option, you have to pay (for) that childcare option and I could not afford (that)" (Camara, age 35).* Many of the parents were looking for free or inexpensive programs that also held extended hours to accommodate the parents' schedules. These types of programs were very difficult to find. Providers also frequently commented on financial concerns as a barrier to accessing preschool programs. As one provider described: *"While McKinney-Vento states that young children should have access to preschool programs, there is not enough funding to provide this service. There are waiting lists for Head Start and Title 1 preschools. The children may still need to wait although they should be able to be immediately enrolled. Preschool services should be available to ALL children."*

In fact, 25% ($N = 243$) of providers endorsed lack of available and affordable slots as a barrier for families in accessing early childhood services. Parents also reflected on this issue, "*They keep you on the waiting list up until they do the lottery over, and then once (they) do it over, even if you're like number two and you didn't get in, you have to reapply all over" (Tiffany, age 23).* Or, as another parent gave voice: *"I've been trying to get my 3-year-old into preschool but the wait list is crazy [long]"* and *"I looked for a preschool closer and... unfortunately it was too late by the time we were looking....most of the [programs] were already full.....they just told me that I have to put – they have to put my child down on a waitlist."* Additionally, when open slots do become available, parents reported that is difficult to find out about them. Furthermore, parents said that when they do find information about programs, it is often too late, or at the wrong time of the year, to enroll their child.

Mobility and communication. Issues associated with mobility also included reference to concerns regarding communication between providers and parents. Providers suggested that it is difficult to locate homeless families, due to a lack of awareness; this concern was endorsed by 17% ($N = 165$) of providers. Providers also reported that it was difficult to maintain contact with families due to parents' lack of phones. The difficulty finding families is more pronounced in rural locations, as illustrated by this provider's comment, "*... There is also a lack of ability to disseminate information regarding programs to families who are isolated geographically."*

Other concerns linked to mobility were voiced directly by parents who had experienced homelessness, including concerns about multiple moves resulting in multiple changes to a child's preschool placement. Several parents provided examples of having to pull their children out of a preschool placement in response to an upcoming move. Only infrequently did a homeless parent seek to find housing near her child's program in order to maintain continuity in the child's education. *"I found out about the school before I found out about the house....wherever they started that's where I wanted to keep him. So I wanted to keep him in that school... I wanted to live in an area that's very close [to that school] and where I didn't have to drive a long ways" (Khloe, age 40).*

In this same vein, families reported challenges with schools not answering their calls or only providing outdated information to families. "*Basically either the information was outdated, or it wasn't for a particular area, or you didn't meet a qualification for this or that. Everything was a runaround" (Erica, age 45).*

Competing demands. Finally, providers as well as parents reported that the experience of homelessness left families with a number of competing demands, limiting their ability to focus on accessing early childhood services. Some of these demands include the challenge of addressing basic needs such as accessing housing, food, and employment to support their families. As one provider stated, families experiencing homelessness often have, "*very chaotic, 'putting out fires' lives and don't often prioritize their child's education when they're concerned about housing, feeding and clothing, and finding a job.*" Parents also substantiated this statement,

Table 5.3 Barriers to accessing early childhood education services

Barriers	NAEHCY findings	Cloudburst findings
Transportation	27% ($N = 262$)	*"So, you can't pay for transportation and you need somewhere you can walk to. These are things you gotta think (about). I gotta get my son somewhere if he gets hurt, I can get up there." (Madison, age 41)*
Lack of available and affordable slots	25% ($N = 243$)	*"I…wanted Head Start because in order to get…a child care option, you have to pay (for) that childcare option and I could not afford (that)." (Camara, age 35)*
Mobility and communication	17% ($N = 559$)	*"I found out about the school before I found out about the house…wherever they started that's where I wanted to keep him. So I wanted to keep him in that school… I wanted to live in an area that's very close [to that school] and where I didn't have to drive a long ways." (Khloe, age 40)*
Competing demands	*"very chaotic, 'putting out fires' lives and don't often prioritize their child's education when they're concerned about housing, feeding and clothing, and finding a job"*	*"I don't know. I don't think I had the time…being in between the shelter and everything else… I wasn't really thinking about preschool. I was thinking about finding a house—a home for us." (Zoe, age 23)*

"I don't know. I don't think I had the time…being in between the shelter and everything else… I wasn't really thinking about preschool. I was thinking about finding a house – a home for us" (Zoe, age 23). (Please see Table 5.3 for a comparison of findings.)

Discussion

This study provides a unique contribution to the literature on access to early childhood services for very young children experiencing homelessness. We acknowledge that the studies are exploratory and the sample size of the Cloudburst study of parental perspectives is decidedly small. However, there was a high degree of corroboration of themes across the two studies, which increases our confidence in the findings. Follow-up research with a larger sample based on the themes emergent from this "small-N" approach may well add to the depth of our understanding.

Themes Emerging from Surveys with Parents and Providers

The surveys of providers and interviews with parents highlight potential policy and practice changes that can help better connect young children experiencing homelessness and their families with early care and education services in their community. Themes that emerged suggest that both providers and parents could benefit from becoming more aware of the availability of early childhood resources, especially when they are new to a community. Both parents and providers can also benefit from policies and practices designed to break down barriers to access and streamline entry into early childhood services, and both would be better served if services in their communities were provided through a cross-sector lens. Additionally, provider surveys highlighted the need for a stronger voice in the service system for attending to the needs of young children experiencing homelessness and their families. Policy and practice recommendations to address the challenges and gaps identified by these studies are provided below.

Increasing Provider Awareness of the Special Needs of Homeless Infants and Toddlers

Providers who responded to the NAEHCY survey felt that there was too little awareness regarding young children's homelessness and that although a sizeable proportion of the homeless population is made up of families with infants, toddlers, and preschool-aged children (Solari et al., 2015). This population is often invisible to the general public as well as many service providers, advocates, and policy makers. This is the case despite the profoundly negative impact that homelessness can have on a very young child's growth, development and learning, (Perlman & Fantuzzo, 2010; Fantuzzo et al., 2013) and even as policies are put into place to use early care and education as an intervention to mitigate the effects that homelessness can have on early brain development and long-term physical well-being. Resources meant to inform the public and others of the plight of homeless families should include clearer reference to newborns and toddlers, and policies and professional resources should address the full scope of individuals experiencing homelessness. Resources exploring and responding to the special needs of infants and young children experiencing homelessness, including training materials, government policy documents, and research publications, must be more widely and visibly disseminated.

Sharing Knowledge About Programs and Services

Findings underscore the recognition that both shelter providers and early childhood educators must do a better job of providing information to families about the various early childhood options available to them. Because the early care and education community does not consistently and actively market their services to homeless families, activities that might publicize early care and education programs locations, what services they provide, and how they can be best accessed, would be of great value. Targeting marketing activities to shelters and housing services providers and others outside of the early care and education service sector would be helpful.

To some degree, this might be linked to increasing participation of the early childhood community in recent HUD-supported efforts to create more comprehensive "Coordinated Entry Systems" in the homeless service provider community. Additionally, with growing focus on quality of care, it would be valuable to have state and local systems for early care and education publicize quality rating efforts so families experiencing homelessness can be aware of where they might find high-quality subsidized care that includes comprehensive services such as that provided by Head Start.

Addressing Systemic Barriers to Help Increase Access and Attendance

Respondents to both the provider survey and parent interviews identified a significant number of barriers to accessing early care and education services. Not only do early care and education programs seem to be hidden to those homeless families who most need to find them, once found, there are myriad challenges to actually using those programs. Clearly, having information about early care and education program locations would ease the search for early childhood services for both homeless services providers and parents. Having accurate and timely information on open slots, waitlists, fees and subsidies, eligibility and residency criteria, and availability of transportation would help parents and providers locate programs that best suit a family's needs for access to early care and education and for sustaining stable enrollment over time. Among changes in programmatic practice that might help to address these concerns are:

- Creating plans in emergency sheltering settings to facilitate smooth transition for children and families into access to early care as well as permanent housing.
- Establishing reimbursement and program "vacancy" rates based on informed estimates of homelessness and mobility in communities, and reserving slots based on those estimates of need to accommodate rolling enrollment of children from homeless families during the school year.
- Ensuring that available information is accurate and up-to-date, while relying on technological and programmatic improvement to decrease the amount of time parents have to invest to craft their own solutions.

Early care programs might also adopt other practices to help mediate the impact of family mobility and decrease logistical barriers to preschool enrollment while in shelter and in transitioning to longer-term housing. The failure of child care and early education programs to adequately meet the individual needs of homeless young children can further exacerbate family instability, resulting in more frequent moves and transitions that can negatively impact a child's ability to learn (Fantuzzo, LeBoeuf, Chen, Rouse, & Culhane, 2012). For parents relocating to a new community, trying to find a high-quality early childhood program with an opening for the particular hours the parent needed and within walking distance can be a significant greater challenge. It is important that shelter staff more actively help families locate early childhood options in the geographic area they are likely to be moving to *after* they exit shelter, rather than focusing only on early care and education options near the shelter. Further, locating affordable housing and quality comprehensive early childhood programs in close proximity could facilitate stable child attendance and create a community of supports for family stability as well. Many parents in this study expressed frustration that they contacted preschool programs too late in the school year to be able to enroll. Although this may be an unavoidable challenge for families who are unsure where they will be residing several months into the future, it can be valuable for housing services staff to encourage them to proactively explore waiting lists and enrollment processes as soon as they know the general location they plan to move to.

Early care programs seeking to act more responsively might:

- Establish policies and practices to target and prioritize homeless families for enrollment and support full inclusion
- Add a priority for homeless or recently homeless families on preschool waiting lists (as is already the case with Head Start programs)
- Explore options for "transporting" slots from one program to another to maintain eligibility across different sites within the same program or system, or assisting families to enroll in similar or appropriate programs near to where they are next moving and/or
- Implement creative strategies to communicate with families, including social media, e-mail, and texting rather than phone calls and mail which are less likely to be useful means of communicating with low-resourced highly mobile families.

Increasing Cross-Sector Collaborations

A high number of participants noted that shelter providers did not discuss preschool as part of the case management provided through emergency shelter. Recognizing that this is a moment in families' lives that is especially challenging and that many children in homeless families experience trauma during these periods of housing instability, (Gewirtz et al., 2008) incorporating discussion of preschool options and mechanisms for accessing preschool as part of a family's crisis services case plan can help to ensure that families are made aware of and can more successfully navigate their way through available options. Including attention to early care and education in housing casework practice can help ensure that the needs of children for quality early care and education and a family's need for a quality care and learning environment for their infants, toddlers, and preschoolers are better met. This, in turn, can support success in parental job search, school enrollment, and engagement in employment.

For families facing complex barriers to self-sufficiency, stability, and wellness, service systems must more actively come together to address those needs appropriately, and must also begin to adopt policies and practices that tie them more closely to one another and to the families they serve. This especially includes the early care and education system which, with the exception of federal Head Start programming, has remained silent on how and with whom it will partner to better meet the needs of this population of young children.

Expanding and Enhancing Training

McKinney–Vento Liaisons, homeless service providers, and early care and education providers are often best positioned to ensure that young children experiencing homelessness are able to access and benefit from the full array of programs and services designed to support healthy child development. Unfortunately, providers often do not receive the training they need to understand and navigate the complex system of services available, identify and refer children who are eligible, and support the children once they are enrolled in programs. Respondents to the NAEHCY provider survey thought that better training was needed to enhance their ability to identify homeless families: *"Identification of children and families experiencing homelessness is huge."* Without open communication with housing and shelter providers and direct outreach to shelters and transitional housing sites where homeless families may be, it is unlikely that McKinney–Vento Liaisons and early care and education and homeless families will easily find one another. There is also a great need for increased understanding of all those in the early childhood and housing services fields of the impact of homelessness on young children and families so that they might better support them and assist in meeting their individual needs. Providers felt that training and technical assistance focused on how to establish networks and relationships with other providers in their community would be helpful in connecting families with services to address their multiple needs. In response to this need, many communities have begun to offer cross-sector training opportunities in which providers from several sectors (e.g., early childhood, housing, education, and child welfare) meet to increase awareness of other sectors and create relationships for working together.

Resources for training that might be more effectively tapped include tools and materials from the Office of Head Start, NAEHCY's early childhood website, the

National Center on Homeless Education, and the U.S. Department of Health and Human Services early childhood website. In addition, memoranda have been created by the Administration for Children and Families for providers that address the importance of connecting young children who are homeless to early intervention, home visiting, and high-quality early childhood education.

Federal and State Leadership, Actions, and Policy Recommendations

At the federal level, Congress and agencies that fund early care and education and homeless service programs can do much more to ensure access to early care and education for children and families experiencing homelessness. Federally funded programs can be targeted toward homeless families by including requirements to prioritize families experiencing homelessness in all federal early childhood programs and initiatives, including child care, the Maternal, Infant, Early Childhood Home Visiting program (MIECHV), federally funded preschool, and Race to the Top Grants. If current capacity cannot be targeted to address the needs of families experiencing homelessness, then increases in federal funding for early care and education programs are needed to provide greater capacity to serve all homeless families.

Many barriers described in both studies could be overcome by extending the full protections afforded through the education subtitle of the McKinney–Vento Homeless Assistance Act to all federally funded early care and education programs. Parents and providers described as challenges the lack of available slots to accommodate all young children in homeless families. Because universal access to early care and education is not yet a reality, McKinney–Vento strategies will need to be adapted to be more appropriate for the limitations of the current early childhood system. Such adaptations could include reserving a small number of program slots for children experiencing homelessness in order to facilitate immediate enrollment, for example. In addition, the US Department of Education could provide clarifying guidance and encouragement for Education for Homeless Children and Youth Program (EHCY) Homeless Liaisons to identify younger children and proactively support families to enroll and participate in early care and education programs and services. In terms of barriers related to transportation, amending the McKinney–Vento Act's Education for Homeless Children and Youth program to strengthen its protections (including transportation) for young children enrolling in early care and education programs would be a huge benefit to families.

To support response to concerns identified by families in this study, the Department of Housing and Urban Development (HUD) should consider the potential impact of policies that could help integrate more thoughtful attention to early care and education access in shelter settings. HUD-funded homeless service programs (and related Homeless Management Information System standards) could consider children as clients separate from their caregivers and appropriately distinguish the child's unique needs in case management plans. Furthermore, programs might be required to facilitate enrollment of young children and families into early care and education programs, report data on rates of such enrollment, and ensure space is provided for early childhood services (e.g., home visiting or early intervention) to provide services to families on site. In this same vein, homeless service agencies might designate a trained staff person to focus on early childhood issues, maintain relationships with early childhood programs in the community, refer children and families to early childhood programs, and assist families in completing required enrollment paperwork.

Through the United States Interagency Council on Homelessness (USICH), HUD, the Department of Health and Human Services (HHS), and the Department of Education, could more actively develop collaborative and complementary policies and approaches to support coordination and integration of early care and education and homeless services at the state and local level. Such policies might require representation from early care and education and McKinney–Vento liaisons on local Continua of Care; representation from the McKinney–Vento State Coordinator on Interagency Coordinating Councils for Early Intervention, Early Childhood State Advisory Councils, MIECHV State Advisories, and state-level interagency councils on homelessness; and inclusion of parents of young children who are homeless and professionals in early care and education on consumer advisory boards for Continua of Care. Additionally, federal agencies could more actively support training and technical assistance opportunities that foster cross-sector collaboration, alignment and sharing of resources, and connection of case management and other direct services to children and families.

States and communities can also play a key role in advancing policies and practices that improve access to early care and education programs for children experiencing homelessness. If they haven't done so already, states might move to align state-funded early care and education programs to the education subtitle of their McKinney–Vento Homeless Assistance programs. Many states fund early care and education programs that are administered outside of school settings, such as early childhood home visiting programs or community-based preschool, and therefore are not compelled to extend the protections afforded to homeless families through the homeless education law. By including requirements for community-based grantees to implement McKinney–Vento practices, states can ensure early care and education programs are utilizing the same definition of homelessness, improve data on this population to inform planning, and create more equitable access to the full array of programs that support the development and school readiness of children experiencing homelessness. Additionally, this would allow states to better leverage the existing McKinney–Vento infrastructure to support alignment of resources horizontally across early care and education programs and vertically between early care and education and K-12 education.

States and communities can reduce system-level barriers to accessing early care and education programs by investing in local community systems development, which could include community-wide common enrollment applications or protocols, central waiting lists, and shared services among early care and education providers. Such intra-system streamlining would make it simpler for families to navigate their choices of services and programs and lay a foundation for more intentional, strategic cross-sector collaboration. States might review funding strategies for early care and education programs and increase incentives for collaboration in a meaningful way while breaking down structures that cause programs in a community to compete for resources.

Conclusion

The experience of homelessness for very young children and their families can have significant effects on each child's long-term educational success and well-being, as well as on family health and stability. Heretofore, this issue, and the related importance of enrollment of young children from homeless families in appropriate early care settings, has received woefully insufficient attention to mitigate negative effects. These companion studies of housing and early childhood providers and of homeless parents highlight the myriad challenges that confront families and young children experiencing homelessness and offer suggestions and opportunities for systems change—grounded in the voices of those most immediately impacted. These voices convey powerful insights that should be heard in shaping policies, programs, and practices better linking the homeless services and early childhood communities to ensure necessary supports and success for all young children and families.

References

Creswell, J. W., & Plano Clark, V. L. P. (2011). *Designing and conducting mixed methods research*. Thousand Oaks, CA: Sage.

Fantuzzo, J., LeBoeuf, W., Brumley, B., & Perlman, S. (2013). A population-based inquiry of homeless episode characteristics and early educational well-being. *Children and Youth Services Review, 35*, 966–972. doi:10.1016/j.childyouth.2013.02.016.

Fantuzzo, J., LeBoeuf, W., Chen, C., Rouse, H., & Culhane, D. (2012). The unique and combined effects of homelessness and school mobility on the educational outcomes of young children. *Educational Researcher, 20*, 1–10. doi:10.3102/0013189X12468210.

Gewirtz, A., Hart-Shegos, E., & Medhanie, A. (2008). Psychosocial status of homeless children and youth in family supportive housing. *American Behavioral Scientist, 51*, 810–823. doi:10.1177/0002764207311989.

Haber, M. G., & Toro, P. A. (2004). Homelessness among families, children, and adolescents: An ecological–developmental perspective. *Clinical Child and Family Psychology Review, 7*, 123–164. doi:10.1023/B:CCFP.0000045124.09503.f1.

Little, M., Shah, R., Vermeulen, M. J., Gorman, A., Dzendoletas, D., & Ray, J. G. (2005). Adverse perinatal outcomes associated with homelessness and substance use in pregnancy. *Canadian Medical Association Journal, 173*(6), 615–618. doi:10.1503/cmaj.050406.

Merrill, R. M., Richards, R., & Sloan, A. (2011). Prenatal maternal stress and physical abuse among homeless women and infant health outcomes in the United States. *Epidemiology Research International*. doi: http://dx.doi.org/10.1155/2011/467265
National Research Council and Institute of Medicine (2000). *From neurons to neighborhoods: The science of early childhood development*. Committee on Integrating the Science of Early Childhood Development. In J. P. Shonkoff, & D. A. Phillips (Eds.), *Board on Children, Youth, and Families, Commission on Behavioral and Social Sciences and Education*. Washington, DC: National Academy Press.
Perlman, S. (2014). *Access to early childhood programs for young children experiencing homelessness: A survey report*. Retrieved from the National Association for the Education of Homeless Children and Youth website: http://www.naehcy.org/sites/default/files/pdf/naehcy-survey-report.pdf
Perlman, S., & Fantuzzo, J. (2010). Timing and influence of early experiences of child maltreatment and homelessness on children's educational well-being. *Children and Youth Services Review*, *32*, 874–883. doi:10.1016/j.childyouth.2010.02.007.
Pope, C., Ziebland, S., & Mays, N. (2000). Qualitative research in health care. Analysing qualitative data. *British Medical Journal*, *320*(7227), 114–116.
Puma, M., Bell, S., Cook, R., Heid, C., Shapiro, G., Broene, P., ... Spier, E. (2010). *Head start impact study* (Final Report). Administration for Children & Families.
Richards, R., Merrill, R. M., & Baksh, L. (2011). Health behaviors and infant health outcomes in homeless pregnant women in the United States. *Pediatrics*, *128*, 438–446.
Solari, C. D., Althoff, S., Bishop, K., Epstein, Z., Morris, S., & Shivji, A. (2015). *2014 Annual homeless assessment report*. U.S. Department of Housing and Urban Development.
Taylor, J., Gibson, B., & Hurd, K. (2015). Parental preschool choices and challenges when young children and their families experience homelessness. *Children and Youth Services Review*, *56*, 68–75. doi:10.1016/j.childyouth.2015.06.010.
U.S. Department of Housing and Urban Development. (2013a). *The 2013 Annual Homeless Assessment Report (AHAR) to Congress*. Retrieved from https://www.hudexchange.info/resources/documents/ahar-2013-part1.pdf
U.S. Department of Housing and Urban Development. (2013b). *Interim Report: Family Options Study*. Retrieved from http://www.huduser.gov/publications/pdf/HUD_503_Family_Options_Study_Interim_Report_v2.pdf

Chapter 6
Interagency Collaboration to Promote Mental Health and Development of Children Experiencing Homelessness

Mary E. Haskett, Jennifer Tisdale, and Amy Leonard Clay

Introduction

As is clear from the introduction to this issue of *Advances in Child and Family Policy and Practice*, children experiencing homelessness warrant the attention of mental health, early childhood, and education professionals. Unfortunately, structural, interpersonal, and individual barriers limit these children's access to appropriate and timely attention from professionals. In addition, services provided to families without homes are not integrated or coordinated between housing agencies or across sectors. Filling service gaps and improving the coordination of mental health and developmental services for children experiencing homelessness was a priority in our community and led to development of Community Action Targeting Children who are Homeless (i.e., Project CATCH) (Donlon, Lake, Pope, Shaw, & Haskett, 2014).

The CATCH vision is that *all families experiencing homelessness in Wake County will have access to a coordinated system of care that nurtures the health, well-being, and success of their children.* The project provides leadership to implement a multitiered system of care by (a) coordinating and integrating shelter and community services for families (community level), (b) changing the structure, policies, and practices of shelters to better support families (shelter level),

---

Author Note: Project CATCH has been funded by grants and support from John Rex Foundation, Wake County Smart Start, The Salvation Army of Wake County, AJ Fletcher Foundation, and United Way of the Greater Triangle, NC.

M.E. Haskett (✉) • A. Leonard Clay
Department of Psychology, North Carolina State University,
Box 7650, Raleigh, NC 27695, USA
e-mail: mehasket@ncsu.edu

J. Tisdale
The Salvation Army, Raleigh, NC, USA

M.E. Haskett (ed.), *Child and Family Well-Being and Homelessness*,
SpringerBriefs in Psychology, DOI 10.1007/978-3-319-50886-3_6

(c) enhancing parenting to strengthen parent–child relationships that can mitigate the potentially harmful impact of homelessness on children (family level), and (d) assessing children's mental health and development to inform referrals for appropriate community services (child level). CATCH is funded by private foundations and state agencies and is staffed by a Coordinator, Outreach Case Manager, Circle of Parents Coordinator, and several part-time employees. It is supported by an advisory group of professionals in young children's mental health, education, business, and homelessness. Herein we describe outcomes after 4 years of operation (2011–2014).

Findings should be considered preliminary because they are based solely on program evaluation data and qualitative observations. We recognize this is not a rigorous evaluation but believe the program should be highlighted because it exemplifies an approach that extends beyond provision of a roof, an approach supported by leaders in the field. Indeed, Project CATCH appears as a model program in the *Services Matter* report by the Bassuk Center on Homeless and Vulnerable Children and Youth (Bassuk, DeCandia, & Richard, 2015), and won national recognition as an exemplary program by the Institute for Children Poverty and Homelessness at the 2016 *Beyond Housing* conference.

Project CATCH Components and Outcomes

Community Level: Coordinate and Integrate Community Services

Rationale. The experience of homelessness can impact multiple domains of parent and child functioning, therefore it is imperative that services are multifaceted and coordinated (Kilmer, Cook, Cursto, Strater, & Haber, 2012). Individual housing programs attempt to link clients to services in the community, but case managers' full caseloads prevent them from accessing services easily and in a coordinated way. Systems-level changes might be more effective when groups of agencies with shared goals join to leverage resources (Harper, Kuperminc, Weaver, Emshoff, & Erickson, 2014). A goal of CATCH is to develop this collective voice to increase the awareness of staff at family-serving agencies and within the wider community about the unique needs of families without homes and to encourage more active and intentional service to these families.

Building a successful coalition. Our housing community includes 11 agencies that provide various forms of emergency and short-term shelter and transitional housing. CATCH brings these diverse programs together to share information relevant to serving families that face homelessness, identify gaps in services, and advocate for increased and improved resources for these families. Structured monthly meetings of CATCH staff and personnel representing all housing partners are the primary method to meet these goals. For this alliance to be most powerful, partner agencies must have regular representation at the meetings.

Table 6.1 Participation in monthly Project CATCH meetings (percent of annual meetings attended)

Housing program	Year 1	Year 2	Year 3	Year 4
Host agency	100	100	100	100
#1	88.8	70	90.9	63.6
#2	66.7	80	100	63.6
#3	33.3	70	90.9	100
#4	66.7	70	45.4	54.4
#5	44.4	60	63.3	54.5
#6	33.3	70	63.6	54.4
#7	33.3	30	45.4	45.4
#8	11.1	80	45.4	9.0
#9	77.8	10	9.0	18.2
#10	33.3	0	0	0
Number of meetings held	9	10	11	11
Number of non-shelter agencies present	10	11	17	19

Attendance records indicate a high level of sustained commitment from most partners (see Table 6.1). Participation remained particularly steady for partners that were active in other components of CATCH, valued the connection to the community of providers, and appreciated the information-sharing related to service challenges and common clients. Relationships with partners seemed to be strengthened by case managers' contacts with housing staff while visiting clients and the introduction of new programming to assist families (e.g., Circle of Parents, described below). In addition, the Coordinator stayed in contact with shelter directors by conducting training sessions on trauma-informed practices and attending partner agency staff meetings to introduce CATCH to newly hired staff and to inform staff about new resources and programs. Only two agencies ceased to attend meetings after the first year. In one case, the simultaneous turnover of leadership at the agency and within CATCH resulted in disruption in the relationship between agencies. At the second site, policies shifted so some CATCH components were available "in house" and staff felt less inclined to attend CATCH meetings. That agency did, however, maintain links to CATCH in other ways.

To gain insight about the value of CATCH meetings after the first year of the program, we surveyed 11 housing partner staff in attendance at a monthly meeting. Respondents had attended an average of 7.3 (range 4–11) monthly meetings over the year, which is quite high given the busy, crisis-oriented work these professionals face. Qualitative and quantitative results are reported below (4 = optimal). Quotes are provided as examples of common replies. These data indicate that shelter staff members experienced a positive impact of CATCH in terms of job satisfaction and effectiveness. The networking opportunities, in particular, were highly valued.

Have the networking and relationship-building opportunities at the CATCH meetings been beneficial to your job effectiveness and satisfaction? Average rating = 3.8

> "There is a supportive, affirming atmosphere which helps us feel we are not out there alone. Many are working cooperatively for the benefit of our most vulnerable, homeless children."

> "Having an opportunity for face to face contact with representatives from other service agencies has been a strategic component in better serving my own clients so they have benefitted from the collaborative work of CATCH."

> "With all the opportunities to strengthen and build community relationships along with the support of the CATCH team, the families and students we serve are able to receive faster, better and more efficient services from the school staff and community."

Do you feel more supported in your work as a result of participation in CATCH meetings? Average rating = 3.4

> "We know that many of our challenges are also shared in other agencies and see the drive in others to help."

> "It is helpful in a sense that sharing common challenges among agencies and populations increases a common feeling of supportiveness."

Has participation in the CATCH meetings provided you with the support needed to remain in your current position at your agency/school? Average rating = 3.3

> "It allows me to re-focus and breathe. The sharing from other providers helps me to remember why I still love my job."

> "... Because this makes our jobs easier in some ways, it has made my current position more enjoyable. Having a partner in the community that cares as deeply about kids experiencing homelessness as [agency] does makes the job much less stressful."

How much are you using the resource information you receive at the CATCH meetings? Average rating = 3.2

> "The guest speakers who have presented during CATCH mtgs have proven to be great resources and aided in serving our clients."

Fostering community partnerships. Although our community is rich in resources, most agencies do not engage in outreach to families in shelters and transitional housing. One of CATCH's greatest benefits is the development of community partnerships with agencies willing to accommodate the unique needs of families without homes. Outreach typically begins with an invitation to a monthly CATCH meeting. There, housing partners learn about the presenting agency's programs and increase awareness about challenges faced by unstably housed families in accessing the agency's services. The meetings often compel agencies to develop ways to increase their efforts to reach homeless families. Over the course of the project there was a nearly 100% increase in number of community partners in attendance (see Table 6.1).

CATCH has developed particularly close working relationships with "fast track" partners that provide basic needs, afterschool programs, health care and mental health treatment, child care and educational programs, parenting support, and services for children with developmental delays. These agencies are aware of our clients' barriers and are willing to overcome them in creative ways. For example, a children's museum offers free annual memberships to CATCH families, thereby enabling children to be exposed to a fun educational experience they might not otherwise have. This museum also offers evening parenting programs specifically for sheltered families, with meals and child care available.

Summary and lessons learned. Housing partner agencies were committed to partnering with other housing providers and carrying out the mission of CATCH. Over the course of 4 years, the depth and breadth of services available to families increased substantially due to pressure exerted through the collective partner agencies. We have learned the value of a central hub for resources, services, and information regarding issues affecting children experiencing homelessness. It should be noted that collaboration among the housing partners and between the housing and community agency partners requires continuous "nurturing" by the CATCH Coordinator and comprises 15–20% of her time. Reevaluation of staff priorities and time commitments might be necessary as we identify and forge a growing number of partnerships to address persistent gaps such as access to tutoring, mental health care for young children, arts programs, adult literacy programs, and transportation.

Shelter Level: Training and Support to Ensure Shelters Are Trauma-Informed

Rationale. Trauma-Informed Care (TIC) is considered best practice in homeless service settings (US Interagency Council on Homelessness, 2010). Agencies that are trauma-informed employ policies and practices grounded in responsiveness to the impact of prior traumatic experiences of clients and creation of an environment that empowers clients and does not further traumatize them (see Guarino, 2014). Because the policies, practices, and culture of many traditional shelters are not optimal for supporting families likely to have experienced trauma (Hooper, Bassuk, & Olivet, 2010), a goal of CATCH is to guide shelters toward providing care and establishing policies that are trauma-informed.

Delivering professional development opportunities. At the outset, we structured our work using the Trauma-Informed Organizational Toolkit developed by the National Center on Family Homelessness (NCFH; Guarino, Soares, Konnath, Clervil, & Bassuk, 2009). In the first year of the project, training in provision of TIC was provided for CATCH staff and housing partner agency personnel through a contract with the NCFH. Training included a web-based overview of the consequences of trauma, a 2-day workshop delivered by the NCFH trainers on trauma-informed best practices (41 people representing 13 agencies attended), and a 2-day training approximately 1 year after the initial training to address questions that arose as agencies began to shift shelter policies and practices to become trauma-informed (67 people representing ten agencies attended). These training sessions were well attended even though there was no external incentive for attendance (e.g., continuing education credits). This speaks to the desire of shelter administrators and staff to provide optimal services to their families.

To reinforce training by national organizations, the CATCH Coordinator provides ongoing support for use of trauma-informed practices. For example, the final agenda item at monthly meetings is a period of self-care exclusively for shelter agency staff. The Coordinator has provided numerous TIC workshops for partner agencies. These sessions are provided to professional staff and evening monitors to increase awareness of trauma with a particular focus on the impact of their own personal experiences and the potential for vicarious trauma. Trainings also have been offered to community partners, including school social workers. Forty-one workshops have been offered for over 600 professionals and 150 parents. Satisfaction surveys were administered at 16 workshops for professional staff, and results indicated a high degree of satisfaction with the content. As shown in Table 6.2, information related to vicarious trauma and self-care was particularly well received. This is not surprising given the heavy stress load carried by the homeless services workforce (Mullen & Leginski, 2010; Olivet, McGraw, Grandin, & Bassuk, 2009). Our results suggest that training that recognizes potential experiences of vicarious trauma of service providers—and provides methods to minimize it—are appreciated by these service providers.

A survey of personnel of 11 partner agencies (seven shelters; four non-shelter partners) was administered after 3 years to examine changes in policies and practices of shelters and priorities for future training provided by CATCH. Respondents agreed (54.5%) or strongly agreed (45.5%) that services had become more trauma-informed and all (100%) had seen improvements in the treatment of clients following the trauma training. Although most respondents (72.7%) reported shelter policies had been altered to be more trauma-informed, three respondents (27.3%) indicated that policies had not changed. Perhaps this was because few

Table 6.2 Ratings of quality of training session content ($N = 16$ workshops)

Workshop content	Mean	Range
Understanding trauma	8.43	8.06–10.00
Impact of trauma: General	8.89	7.87–9.71
Impact of trauma on the brain	7.85	7.05–9.75
Providing trauma-informed care	8.55	8.40–8.60
Vicarious trauma	9.00	8.36–9.75
Importance of self-care	8.74	6.94–9.57
Adjusting the intake process	7.63	6.90–8.40
Role play exercise	8.30	6.93–9.85

Note. A rating of 1 = low quality content; 10 = high quality content

administrators and other decision-makers at those particular shelters had attended training. Respondents expressed strong (63.6%) or very strong (36.4%) interest in further training. High turnover among shelter staff and the intensity of work in shelter settings (Olivet et al., 2009) likely contributed to the desire for continued training.

Summary and lessons learned. On a positive note, training in trauma-informed care was well attended and staff reported changes in shelter practices. Attending a training session can be a good first step in the change process, but systems-level shifts will occur only if knowledge of TIC is consistently practiced and TIC goals are embraced by administrators (Guarino, 2014). Moving forward, we will seek greater agency commitment to systemic change and we will emphasize sustainability of trauma-informed care by internalization of TIC practices. We also will consider ways to use the NCFH Toolkit more intentionally and create the means to assess change in practices and cultural shift of organizations. A field-tested and validated version of an agency self-assessment (the Trauma Informed Care Organizational Meter) was recently released for this purpose by the Center for Social Innovation (Bassuk, Unick, Paquette, & Richard, 2016).

Family Level: Services to Enhance Parenting and the Parent–Child Relationship

Rationale. The majority of children who are homeless are young, with about 50% under the age of 5 years (Bassuk, DeCandia, Beach, & Berman, 2014); therefore, a priority was placed on promoting children's development and positive social–emotional adjustment indirectly, by supporting parents in their caregiving role. Positive parenting contributes to resilience of children exposed to early challenges, including homelessness (Cutuli & Herbers, 2014; Miliotis, Sesma, & Masten, 1999), but many parents who are homeless do not consistently provide safe and positive parenting (e.g., Lee et al., 2010) and many experience high stress in the parenting role (Holtrop, McNeil, & McWey, 2015). To enhance parenting skills, lower parenting stress, and support healthy parent/child relationships of families in shelters, CATCH facilitates on-site parenting programs. We have been strategic in promoting evidence-based or research-informed programs. Because needs of families in shelters are highly diverse and the shelters differ in mission, structure, and clients, a variety of programs have been introduced. It was critical that each intervention would be feasible within constraints of the shelter setting, was consistent with trauma-informed practices, and was culturally sensitive.

Services delivered by CATCH. Most of the interventions introduced by CATCH have been delivered to parents through community agency partnerships. An exception was Theraplay, an attachment-based therapy for building and enhancing attachment, self-esteem, trust in others, and "joyful engagement" among family members (Wettig, Coleman, & Geider, 2011). According to the California

Evidence-Based Clearinghouse (CEBC) for Child Welfare, there is “promising research evidence” for Theraplay in the area of infant and toddler mental health. There is some research to support the benefits of Theraplay for children’s communication skills and trust (Wettig et al., 2011) and behavioral functioning (Weir et al., 2013).

A CATCH case manager obtained certification to provide Theraplay for parents at the CATCH host agency and a social work intern served as co-therapist. Seven mothers of children 2–4 years of age enrolled in the intervention, which took place in six group sessions over 8 months. One mother dropped out after the first session but all others completed the sessions, yielding a very high retention rate. No outcome data were collected but the therapists provided anecdotal reports of changes over time. During the first session, families arrived late and reluctantly; over the course of the intervention, they began to come early and remained together well after the session ended. In the first session only one mother engaged with her child; the other children were drawn to her and readily left their own mothers to interact with her. Other mothers were passive and unengaged, and did not attempt to interact with their own children. The therapists decided to have a gentle conversation with each mother individually about the importance of play and the value of touch to prepare them to benefit from Theraplay. They found parents didn’t have basic engagement skills or understand the benefits of play, so they taught mothers simple games. In later sessions, mothers and children were observed smiling and laughing together and children increasingly were apt to climb into their mother’s lap. Therapists noticed that mothers began to use songs learned in the group to gain their child’s attention outside group. Parents not in the group asked to participate and older children approached the therapist to ask if they could have a group. When the intern’s placement ended, the primary therapist was unable to continue to offer Theraplay due to other work responsibilities. Because sustainability of programs presented a challenge due to case managers’ limited time to provide direct services, CATCH staff made the decision to focus on (a) pursuit of special funding to support direct services by hiring treatment providers and (b) building collaborations to capitalize on existing community agencies’ expertise and programs to serve families on-site in shelters.

Although there are some discrepancies in findings across studies, research indicates that many individuals experiencing homelessness report social isolation and lack of emotional and instrumental support (Eyrich, Pollio, & North, 2003; Zugazaga, 2008). The important role of social support for positive parenting has been demonstrated in several studies (e.g., Heberle, Krill, Briggs-Gowan, & Cater, 2015) and support might serve as a protective factor against depression and anxiety for homeless adults (Fitzpatrick, 2014). To increase social support among parents in housing partner agencies, the CATCH host agency facilitated Circle of Parents in four housing programs. Circle of Parents is a mutual self-help support group model developed to prevent child abuse and neglect and strengthen families (Circle of Parents, 2014). Parents participate in weekly group meetings to share information, develop and practice new parenting skills, learn about community resources, and give and receive support. Groups are parent-led with the support of a trained group facilitator and children's programs operate concurrent with parent meetings. Circle of Parents was reviewed by the CEBC but evidence to support the program was insufficient to apply a rating. At the end of the first year of Circle of Parents, the groups had included a total of 281 parents (211 women, seven men) and 301 children.

To formally evaluate the Circle of Parents groups, investigators administered the Protective Factors Survey (PFS) to 39 parents who participated in the groups and 41 parents who resided in shelters without groups; the PFS was administered at the start of Circle of Parents groups and again 4 months later (Haskett et al., 2017). Parents who attended groups also completed a survey of satisfaction. Results indicated that groups generally were feasible in shelters and Circle of Parents was highly acceptable to parents. However, analyses indicated no significant effects in terms of enhanced protective factors. One explanation for this finding is that 4 months of involvement in Circle of Parents groups was not adequate to result in significant change in protective factors.

Services delivered by community partners. The first collaboration between CATCH and a community partner to support parenting was developed with our Head Start agency. The intervention provided was Raising a Thinking Child (Shure & DiGeronimo, 1996), a program based on the I Can Problem Solve curriculum (Spivack & Shure, 1989) designed to help children develop problem-solving skills to reduce behavior problems. I Can Problem Solve has been rated "promising" by the CEBC in the area of disruptive behavior treatment. The 10-week groups, led by a Head Start employee who was co-located in four shelters, were open to parents in any housing program. Approximately 35 parents participated, with a retention rate of 95%, which is incredibly high for a parenting group and especially impressive given the transient nature of the population. The practitioner who led groups noted that no modifications were necessary to conduct the groups in the shelter setting. Unfortunately, there were no resources to administer outcome or satisfaction measures. Based on anecdotal observations, the group leader reported that the group was successful in creating a "community atmosphere" for families. Parents gained trust in each other and began to use each other as resources. Parents were able to teach their children to use problem-solving vocabulary, empathize with others, and see things from the point of view of others. Parents gave the group leader examples of how they had learned to calm down and think before they reacted to challenging child behaviors.

A second parenting program offered via CATCH collaborations with community partners is Triple P-Positive Parenting Program, an evidence-based tiered suite of parenting interventions rated as "supported" for parent training by the CEBC. Triple P is associated with reductions in child behavior problems and increases in positive parenting as well as reductions in child abuse risk (e.g., Prinz, Sanders, Shapiro, Whitaker, & Lutzker, 2009; Sanders, Baker, & Turner, 2012). A recent study showed that women residing in shelters found Triple P materials to be relevant, and the intervention delivery methods to be acceptable (Wessels & Ward, 2016). Our public school system obtained funding to implement Triple P by training the existing workforce in more than 25 agencies to deliver Triple P to community parents. The school system recognized the central role of Project CATCH in our community and trained providers to deliver Triple P to families in CATCH housing partner agencies.

To date, the providers have offered Triple P Seminars on general positive parenting approaches and Discussion Groups on specific child-management challenges (e.g., disobedience) to parents in almost all housing partner agencies. Providers are also present at some of the shelters to be available for individual parenting support, but parents have been a bit slower to take advantage of individual sessions compared to their willingness to attend groups. This was consistent with the findings of Wessels and Ward (2016) who reported that mothers in shelters rated group delivery of Triple P more acceptable than individual delivery. In addition to the two providers hired by the school system to serve families in shelters, two other agencies co-locate staff in shelters to provide Triple P and staff at several shelters have been trained to deliver Triple P. This speaks to the success of CATCH at increasing awareness of community agencies about the needs of families without homes and encouraging those agencies to extend services to sheltered families. The CATCH Coordinator serves on the Steering Committee for the Triple P initiative, which illustrates the central role of CATCH in community initiatives.

Client satisfaction surveys are administered to parents after 90-min Triple P Seminars. Satisfaction data were available for 181 parents who attended one of 25 seminars held in one of eight housing programs. As shown in Table 6.3, there was consistently high satisfaction among the parents for all aspects of the seminars. On a seven-point scale, ratings were above 6.0 on every aspect. For example, parents indicated they were highly likely to use the parenting advice they received ($M = 6.73$; SD = 0.62). Collaboration with a doctoral student at a local university will allow CATCH to examine effects of Triple P Discussion Groups with parents in shelters; that study will include a wait-list control group of parents experiencing homelessness.

Table 6.3 Mean (SD) parent satisfaction ratings for Triple P seminars ($N = 181$)

Satisfaction item	Mean rating (SD)	Range
How would you rate the quality of the seminar presentation?	6.74 (0.58)	5–7
Did the seminar provide sufficient opportunities for questions?	6.73 (0.62)	4–7
Was the seminar interesting to you?	6.65 (0.77)	3–7
Did the presenter use clear examples to illustrate parenting issues?	6.84 (0.43)	5–7
Did the presenter provide clear explanations?	6.85 (0.40)	5–7
Did you gain sufficient knowledge to implement the parenting advice you heard about?	6.70 (0.64)	3–7
Overall, how would you rate the content of the seminar?	6.79 (0.53)	4–7
Was the seminar helpful in gaining an understanding of what you can do to help your child learn new skills and behavior?	6.70 (0.63)	3–7
Was the parenting tip sheet you received useful?	6.71 (0.62)	3–7
Do you intend to implement the parenting advice you received?	6.73 (0.62)	4–7

Note. A rating of 1 = low satisfaction; 7 = high satisfaction

Summary and lessons learned. Our experience with a variety of parenting interventions indicates that programs are feasible in shelters with minor modifications, *if* resources are sufficient to staff the programs. Two programs were discontinued when funding ended (Raising a Thinking Child) or staffing changed (Theraplay). Consistent with the literature on parenting support provided in shelters (Haskett, Loehman, & Burkhart, 2014), parents in our housing partner agencies welcomed the opportunity to engage in parenting support and rated the programs very positively. Anecdotally, they were more drawn to support provided in a group setting and were less responsive to offers for individual parenting support. As Triple P becomes more embedded in shelters, we expect that acceptability of individual support will increase. Although parents were highly satisfied with the group interventions offered, the evaluation of Circle of Parents did not indicate significant improvements in protective factors. Continued outcome research is needed to identify effective supports for parents experiencing homelessness. Conducting methodologically sound evaluations of these programs is a significant challenge (Gewirtz, Burkhart, Loehman, & Haukebo, 2014).

Child Level: Assess Children's Functioning and Refer to Appropriate Services

Rationale. Research indicates that children without homes are much more likely than children in stable housing to have developmental delays, and they exhibit a high rate of mental health challenges (Bassuk, Richard, & Tsertsvadze, 2015; Park, Fertig, & Allison, 2011). Thus, developmental and mental health screening of these children should be a priority; however, children experiencing homelessness are not routinely screened or identified for services (see DeCandia et al chapter in this Brief). Because none of the housing programs in our community were equipped to conduct these evaluations, child screenings and subsequent case management were a priority task for CATCH.

Screening and referrals. During the screening, a psychosocial interview is conducted with parents, followed by administration of the Brigance Early Childhood Screen II (Brigance, 2010) to assess the developmental status of children ages birth to 1st grade. To assess children's social–emotional adjustment, parents of children birth to 5 years complete the Ages and Stages Questionnaire: Social Emotional form (Squires, Bricker, & Twombly, 2002) and parents of older children complete the Eyberg Child Behavior Inventory (Eyberg & Pincus, 1999) and/or Strengths and Difficulties Questionnaire (Goodman, 1997). Collateral information such as medical and school records are obtained and reviewed. Finally, family and child strengths and needs are identified and appropriate referrals for services are made. Referrals for CATCH clients are prioritized by many of our fast track partners to reduce wait times. A database is used to track referrals and the services children receive; this allows the case manager to follow families and facilitate connection with resources as needed.

After 4 years, 1393 children (754 aged birth to 5; 639 over age five) had been referred to CATCH and over 1900 services had been provided to those children. On average, 84% of children referred for screening received an intervention/service after referral. Many parents contact their case manager to seek referrals for assistance well after leaving shelters. This speaks to the value of providing a continuum of care for families and to the importance of case management for children. CATCH case managers often are the only point of contact families have with service providers after they leave the shelter. A study based on 328 young children screened by CATCH provides strong justification for the screening component (Haskett, Armstrong, & Tisdale, 2015). Specifically, analysis of the children's Brigance scores indicated the mean level of functioning for the sheltered children was significantly below the mean score for the norming sample. Parents of 24.6% of the children indicated significant concerns related to their child's mental health (i.e., ASQ scores were above the threshold for a referral for mental health services) (Haskett et al., 2015).

Community agencies provide most of the direct services to CATCH children after a referral from the CATCH case manager. The only direct intervention provided to children by CATCH is Physical and Emotional Awareness for Children who are Homeless (PEACH), a 16-session curriculum developed by the National Center on Family Homelessness to teach groups of young children about good nutrition, physical activity, and how to deal with the emotional stress of being homeless. To date, PEACH has been conducted in three CATCH partner shelters by the CATCH case manager. In each series there were about eight children ages 3–6 enrolled. PEACH also has been conducted during Circle of Parents groups in several shelters. PEACH is appealing for shelter providers because it is enjoyed by young children and is easily implemented by community volunteers; however, no outcome data have yet been collected to evaluate the effect of PEACH.

Summary and lessons learned. A large proportion of children referred for screening and case management were under the age of five, which reflects the fact that children five and younger are overrepresented nationally in the population of children experiencing homelessness. The necessity for this component of CATCH is clear in the high number of children referred for screening and the proportion who received services. The need is further underscored by the results of screenings that indicated a high potential for developmental delays and social–emotional challenges among children experiencing homelessness. Given this evidence of high risk, we will expand screening services (as described below) to reach a larger proportion of children without homes in our community.

Overall Project Evaluation

As noted above, the Coordinator administered a survey to representatives of 11 partner agencies in attendance at a monthly meeting at the end of three years of CATCH. When asked open-ended questions about how CATCH had impacted their agency, the wider community, and children and families they served, respondents focused on the benefits of increased connections across agencies, resource sharing, and improvements in services they provided to families. Verbatim quotes from providers are provided below to illustrate these reported benefits.

> "Without the support of CATCH, more families will fall further into crisis... [CATCH is] the only community group to proactively provide assessments and assistance to non-school aged children in transition. With this proactive approach to intervening early, the child is likely to find more success in the school setting and, ultimately, in life than if CATCH was not involved."

> "CATCH has impacted the community in a positive way by linking so many resources and continuing to address the needs of children and families experiencing homelessness...".

> "CATCH has connected us [a shelter program] with the community."

> "We [a shelter program] are so different now and can use data to help guide us in decisions and programming."

> "CATCH has positively impacted the families and children in our residential program by being able to connect to another community agency that can assist and support them throughout their stay and after they exit the shelter."

Respondents also were asked to rank-order four foundational CATCH services in order of importance in meeting the needs of their families. The services were (a) development screenings and case management, (b) opportunity to share resources, (c) collaboration across agencies, and (d) training in trauma-informed care. Findings indicated that the most critical service was child developmental screenings with case management; 10 (90.9%) ranked this component as the first or second most critical service. Indeed, this was the most pressing need when the community initially identified gaps in services for children experiencing homelessness. Findings with respect to the other components of CATCH were somewhat mixed. The opportunity to share resources and to collaborate across shelter partners and other agencies were ranked highly by five (45%) of respondents but three (27%) indicated those opportunities were least critical. Training in trauma was considered most critical by one respondent, with the remaining ranking it the least critical. This may be due to the fact that training was not considered essential to assisting their children.

Using a scale of 1 = *Disagree Strongly* to 4 = *Agree Strongly*, respondents rated their level of agreement with four statements related to CATCH. They assigned a mean rating of 3.82 to the statement "CATCH provides strong community support and collaboration among agencies and fosters beneficial partnerships with community organizations." They assigned a mean rating of 3.54 to the statement "Without CATCH's services, children would be at risk of falling through the cracks and not being connected to services." In response to the item, "CATCH provides a valuable community service for our agency and the children we serve," respondents provided a mean rating of 3.60. Respondents provided a mean rating of 3.70 to the statement "My agency would like CATCH to continue serving in the same capacity as a collaborative partner."

Conclusions, Future Directions, and Policy Implications

This initial program evaluation of CATCH provides support for continuation of the project. The collaboration has been successful as partners and agencies rally around the collective goal of ensuring the needs of children experiencing homelessness are met. Partner agency staff believe the collaborative has strengthened and expanded service delivery and access to resources within the community, beyond what might have been accomplished in four years if agencies operated alone as they had done previously. It likely is a cost savings for CATCH case managers to serve children who are homeless across housing agencies rather than each agency hiring their own child case manager. Most housing partner agencies have embraced the parenting programs initiated in their agencies with the support and coordination of CATCH, and parents have responded positively. Finally, personnel at partner agencies value the training in trauma-informed care and report increased knowledge and changes in practices at their housing programs that are consistent with a trauma-informed approach to serving families. Institutional policy change has been more challenging and gradual, which is consistent with research on the pace of cultural change in complex organizations (Thomas & Amber, 2014). We believe some of the keys to success of CATCH are dual engagement from both administrative/leadership levels and direct service personnel; consistent contact with agencies through face-to-face interaction; timely provision of quality services; developing a sense of comradery and trust; and resource sharing towards a common end—to improve the lives of underserved, deeply valued children.

Future plans. Sustainability, growth of the collaborative, and formal outcome evaluation are current goals. In terms of sustainability, diversifying sources of funding will be critical and several avenues for creative funding are being pursued. With respect to expansion of services, we will work to increase the percentage of children in shelters who are screened by CATCH and we recently secured funding through a collective impact grant to reach families living in motels and hotels. Research on collaboration is fraught with methodological challenges (Gabriel, 2000) and we continue to work toward increasing the sophistication of data collection to document process and outcomes of CATCH. Recently, focus has broadened to extending the "reach" of CATCH. Child screening data are being used to support advocacy efforts at the state level to increase identification of young homeless children at risk for delays and to increase the rate of referrals for determination of eligibility for early intervention services.

Policy implications. Outcomes of CATCH suggest that intensive collaboration among housing programs and between the housing community and larger community of family-serving agencies is feasible and valuable. Growing rates of family homelessness and the pressing needs of children in these families warrant policies that encourage agency cooperation and stipulation that children who are homeless are prioritized for services. The National Center on Early Head Start Child Care Partnerships, jointly funded by the Office of Head Start and the Office of Child Care, encourages development of formal partnerships between Early Head Start and child care programs. Such partnerships could be expanded to include housing providers, McKinney–Vento coordinators, and early intervention agencies. Funders of programs to support homeless families should actively encourage collaboration to achieve system-wide goals; initiatives to promote collective impact provide an excellent foundation for such cross-sector projects. Although there was evidence of individual differences in functioning among our children, results of screenings point to high risk for delays and social–emotional difficulties among children experiencing homelessness. These findings are consistent with the existing literature; together, this body of research could be used as a basis to advocate for systematic eligibility screening of homeless children for early intervention. Advocates in Pennsylvania were recently successful in this endeavor (PA House bill 2204, i.e., the "Yay Babies" campaign) and we are conducting similar work in our state. Finally, our results indicate that many parents experiencing homelessness are eager to receive support for parenting. These parents should have greater access to parenting support and the Maternal, Infant, and Early Childhood Home Visiting program established in 2010 could be a source of funding to promote positive parenting and reduce early social–emotional–behavioral challenges of young homeless children.

References

Bassuk, E. L., DeCandia, C. J., & Richard, M. K. (2015). *Services matter: How housing and services can end family homelessness*. Needham, MA: The Bassuk Center.

Bassuk, E. L., Richard, M. K., & Tsertsvadze, A. (2015). The prevalence of mental illness in homeless children: A systematic review and meta-analysis. *Journal of the American Academy of Child and Adolescent Psychiatry*, *54*, 86–96. doi:10.1016/j.jaac.2014.11.008.

Bassuk, E. L., DeCandia, C. J., Beach, C. A., & Berman, F. (2014). *America's youngest outcasts: A report card on child homelessness*. Waltham, MA: The National Center on Family Homelessness at American Institutes for Research. Retrieved from www.homelesschildrenamerica.org

Bassuk, E. L., Unick, J., Paquette, K., Richard, M. K. (2016). Developing an Instrument to Measure Organizational Trauma-Informed Care in Human Services: *The TICOMETER*. *Psychology of Violence*, Advance online posting, January 21 doi.org/10.1037/vio0000030

Brigance, A. H. (2010). *Brigance Early Childhood Screen II*. North Billerica, MA: Curriculum Associates.

Circle of Parents. (2014). Retrieved from www.circleofparents.org

Cutuli, J. J., & Herbers, J. E. (2014). Promoting resilience for children who experience family homelessness: Opportunities to encourage developmental competence. *Cityscape*, *16*, 113–140.

Donlon, P., Lake, J., Pope, E., Shaw, C., & Haskett, M. E. (2014). Community Action Targeting Children who are Homeless (CATCH): Addressing the mental health and developmental needs of children experiencing homelessness. *Families in Society*, *95*, 163–170. doi:10.1606/1044-3894.2014.95.21.

Eyberg, S. M., & Pincus, D. (1999). *Eyberg child behavior inventory and Sutter-Eyberg student behavior inventory: Professional manual*. Odessa, FL: Psychological Assessment Resources.

Eyrich, K. M., Pollio, D. E., & North, C. S. (2003). An exploration of alienation and replacement theories of social support in homelessness. *Social Work Research*, *27*, 222–231. doi:10.1093/swr/27.4.222.

Fitzpatrick, K. M. (2014). How positive is their future? Assessing the role of optimism and social support in understanding mental health symptomatology among homeless adults. *Stress and Health* . doi:10.1002/smi.2676.Online first posting, April 1, 2016

Gabriel, R. M. (2000). Methodological challenges in evaluating community partnerships & coalitions: Still crazy after all these years. *Journal of Community Psychology*, *28*, 339–352. doi:10.1002/(SICI)1520-6629(200005)28:3<339::AID-JCOP8>3.0.CO;2-9.

Gewirtz, A., Burkhart, K., Loehman, J., & Haukebo, B. (2014). Research on programs designed to support positive parenting. In M. E. Haskett, S. Perlman, & B. Cowan (Eds.), *Supporting families experiencing homelessness: Current practices and future directions* (pp. 57–77). New York: Springer.

Goodman, R. (1997). The strengths and difficulties questionnaire: A research note. *Journal of Child Psychology and Psychiatry*, *38*, 581–586. doi:10.1111/j.1469-7610.1997.tb01545.x.

Guarino, K. M. (2014). Trauma-informed care for families experiencing homelessness. In M. E. Haskett, S. Perlman, & B. Cowan (Eds.), *Supporting families experiencing homelessness: Current practices and future directions*. New York: Springer.

Guarino, K., Soares, P., Konnath, K., Clervil, R., & Bassuk, E. (2009). *Trauma-informed organizational toolkit*. Rockville, MD: Center for Mental Health Services, Substance Abuse and Mental Health Services Administration, and the Daniels Fund, the National Child Traumatic Stress Network, and the W.K. Kellogg Foundation. Retrieved from http://www.familyhomelessness.org/media/90.pdf.

Harper, C. R., Kuperminc, G. P., Weaver, S. R., Emshoff, J., & Erickson, S. (2014). Leveraged resources and systems changes in community collaboration. *American Journal of Community Psychology*, *54*, 348–357. doi:10.1007/s10464-014-9678-7.

Haskett, M. E., Armstrong, J., & Tisdale, J. (2015). Developmental status and social-emotional functioning of young children experiencing homelessness. *Early Childhood Education Journal*, *44*(2), 119–125 Online first posting, February 2015. doi:10.1007/s10643-015-0691-8.

Haskett, M. E., Loehman, J., & Burkhart, K. (2014). Parenting interventions in shelters: A qualitative systematic review of the literature. Child & Family Social Work. 21(3), 272–282. doi:10.1111/cfs.12147. Retrieved March 2014.

Haskett, M. E., Okoniewski, K. C., Armstrong, J., Galanti, S., Lowder, E., Loehman, J., & Lanier, P. J. (2017). Feasibility, acceptability, and effects of a peer support group to prevent child maltreatment among parents experiencing homelessness. *Children and Youth Services Review*. *73*, 187–196. doi:10.1016/j.childyouth.2016.12.012.

Heberle, A. E., Krill, S. C., Briggs-Gowan, M. J., & Cater, A. S. (2015). Predicting externalizing and internalizing behavior in kindergarten: Examining the buffering role of early social support. *Journal of Clinical Child & Adolescent Psychology*, *44*, 640–654. doi:10.1080/15374416.2014.886254.

Holtrop, K., McNeil, S., & McWey, L. M. (2015). "It's a struggle but I can do it. I'm doing it for me and my kids": The psychosocial characteristics and life experiences of at-risk homeless parents in transitional housing. *Journal of Marital and Family Therapy*, *41*, 177–191. doi:10.1111/jmft.12050.

Hooper, E., Bassuk, E., & Olivet, J. (2010). Shelter from the storm: Trauma-informed care in homelessness service settings. *The Open Health Services and Policy Journal*, *3*, 80–100. doi:10.2174/1874924001003010080.

Kilmer, R. P., Cook, J. R., Cursto, C., Strater, K. P., & Haber, M. G. (2012). Understanding the ecology and development of children and families experiencing homelessness: Implications for practice, supportive services, and policy. *American Journal of Orthopsychiatry*, *82*, 389–401. doi:10.1111/j.1939-0025.2012.01160.x.

Lee, S. S., August, G. J., Gewirtz, A. H., Klimes-Dougan, B., Bloomquist, M. L., & Realmuto, G. M. (2010). Identifying unmet mental health needs in children of formerly homeless mothers living in a supportive housing community sector of care. *Journal of Abnormal Child Psychology*, *38*, 421–432.

Miliotis, D., Sesma, A., & Masten, A. S. (1999). Parenting as a protective process for school success in children from homeless families. *Early Education and Development*, *10*, 111–133. doi:10.1207/s15566935eed1002_2.

Mullen, J., & Leginski, W. (2010). Building the capacity of the homeless service workforce. *The Open Health Services and Policy Journal, 2*, 101–110. Retrieved from http://www.nhchc.org/wp-content/uploads/2013/01/Winter2013HealingHands.pdf
Olivet, J., McGraw, S., Grandin, M., & Bassuk, E. (2009). *Staffing challenges and strategies for organizations serving individuals who have experienced chronic homelessness*. Rockville, MD: Center for Mental Health Services, Substance Abuse and Mental Health Services Administration.
Park, J., Fertig, A., & Allison, P. (2011). Physical and mental health, cognitive development, and health care use by housing status of low-income young children in 20 American cities: A prospective cohort study. *American Journal of Public Health, 101*, S255–S261. doi:10.2105/AJPH.2010.300098.
Prinz, R., Sanders, M. R., Shapiro, C. J., Whitaker, D. J., & Lutzker, J. R. (2009). Population-based prevention of child maltreatment: The U.S. Triple P system population trial. *Prevention Science, 10*, 1–12. doi:10.1007/s11121-009-0123-3.
Sanders, M. R., Baker, S., & Turner, K. (2012). A randomized controlled trial evaluating the efficacy of Triple P online with parents of children with early-onset conduct problems. *Behaviour Research and Therapy, 50*, 675–684. doi:10.1016/j.brat.2012.07.004.
Shure, M., & DiGeronimo, T. F. (1996). *Raising a thinking child*. New York, NY: Pocket Books.
Spivack, G., & Shure, M. (1989). Interpersonal Cognitive Problem Solving (ICPS): A competence-building primary prevention program. *Prevention in Human Services, 6*, 151–117. doi:10.1080/10852358909511187.
Squires, J., Bricker, D., & Twombly, L. (2002). *Ages and stages questionnaires: Social-emotional*. Baltimore, MD: Brookes Publishing.
Thomas, P., & Amber, S. (2014). Organizational change tactics: The evidence base in the literature. *Journal of Evidence-Based Social Work, 11*, 498–450. doi:10.1080/15433714.2013.831006.
US Interagency Council on Homelessness (2010). Opening doors: Federal strategic plan to prevent and end homelessness. Retrieved from http://www.usich.gov/PDF/OpeningDoors_2010_FSPPreventEndHomeless.pdf
Weir, K., Lee, S., Canosa, P., Rodrigues, N., McWilliams, M., & Parker, L. (2013). Whole family theraplay: Integrating family systems theory and theraplay to treat adoptive families. *Adoption Quarterly, 16*, 175–200. doi:10.1080/10926755.2013.844216.
Wessels, I., & Ward, C. (2016). Battered women and parenting: Acceptability of an evidence-based parenting programme to women in shelters. *Journal of Child & Adolescent Mental Health, 28*, 21–31. doi:10.2989/17280583.2015.1132425.
Wettig, H. G., Coleman, A. R., & Geider, F. J. (2011). Evaluating the effectiveness of Theraplay in treating shy, socially withdrawn children. *International Journal of Play Therapy, 20*, 26–37. doi:10.1037/a0022666.
Zugazaga, C. B. (2008). Understanding social support of the homeless: A comparison of single men, single women, and women with children. *Families in Society: The Journal of Contemporary Social Services, 89*, 447–455. doi:10.1606/1044-3894.3770.

Chapter 7
A Safe, Stable Place to Call Home: Policy Implications and Next Steps to Address Family Homelessness

Preston A. Britner and Anne F. Farrell

Introduction

In 2010, the Obama administration launched the *Opening Doors* campaign, and with it, announced a plan to end homelessness among children, youth, and families (U.S. Interagency Council on Homelessness (USICH), 2015). The *Opening Doors* plan engages a guiding vision, "...no one should be without a safe, stable place to call home," and sets forth the objective that every community have in place systematic responses to prevent homelessness and ensure that homeless episodes are rare, short, and nonrecurring. The plan calls for four essential capacities: prompt, effective means to identify individuals at risk; intervention to prevent the loss of housing and avert homelessness; when homelessness cannot be avoided, immediate access to shelter and crisis supports while permanent housing and related supports are secured; and, rapid connection to supports that are tailored to families' unique needs and strengths, with the ultimate objective of securing permanent, safe, stable housing. An unvoiced assumption is the notion that government's role in ensuring safe, affordable housing may "yield social benefits" (Leventhal & Newman, 2010, p. 1166) and thus might address persisting gaps in educational, vocational, and income attainment among families caught in intergenerational cycles of poverty, among whom racial and ethnic minorities are disproportionately represented.

Author Note: The authors express their appreciation to Amy Dworsky, Ph.D., Chapin Hall at the University of Chicago, for comments on an earlier version of this chapter.

P.A. Britner (✉)
Department of Human Development and Family Studies, University of Connecticut,
348 Mansfield Road, U-1058, Storrs, CT 06269, USA
e-mail: Preston.Britner@UConn.edu

A.F. Farrell
Chapin Hall at the University of Chicago, Chicago, IL, USA

M.E. Haskett (ed.), *Child and Family Well-Being and Homelessness*,
SpringerBriefs in Psychology, DOI 10.1007/978-3-319-50886-3_7

The bold vision that is *Opening Doors*, specifically, a vision to end homelessness, compels the prompt application of an emerging corpus of scholarship and valuable field experiences to change policies and practices that create and perpetuate family homelessness, and its attendant causes and consequences. Whereas efforts to prevent homelessness increased significantly under the Homeless Prevention and Rapid Rehousing Program as part of the American Recovery and Reinvestment Act of 2009 (e.g., $1.5 billion in funding), families appear to be an increasingly visible segment of the homeless population and tend to be involved in multiple public systems (Grant, Gracy, Goldsmith, Shapiro, & Redlener, 2013). Nevertheless, in a systematic review of the literature, Bassuk, DeCandia, Tsertsvadze, and Richard (2014) found few rigorous studies upon which to draw any significant conclusions about "what works" to end family homelessness. The articles in this issue of *Advances in Child and Family Policy and Practice* do more than remind us that family homelessness is too common; these authors contribute policy-relevant knowledge with actionable implications. Taken together, these authors identify important empirical findings about the characteristics and needs of homeless families, as well as their responses to assessment, engagement, service, and coordination practices currently in place. In this synthesis, we recap some of the key findings and highlight key policy implications. We interweave the implications within the text and further underscore actionable, pragmatic policy and practice considerations in "pullout" text boxes.

Assessment Is a Relational Activity

DeCandia, Bassuk, and Richard (this issue) provide a vital look at the relevance and nature of assessment practices when homeless families enter shelter. The authors explain the importance of assessing family members to identify strengths and needs and determine an appropriate case plan. They describe assessment as a "relational activity" between providers and clients. We agree. In our own research on supportive housing for families involved in child welfare (e.g., Farrell, Britner, Guzzardo, & Goodrich, 2010), we have seen strong intake and assessment procedures (including motivational interviewing and other techniques designed to involve families as active partners) to be critically important to engagement in services.

DeCandia et al. note that the U.S. Department of Housing and Urban Development required each Continuum of Care (CoC) to develop a coordinated assessment tool to assess eligibility, match to housing options, and guide referrals. With limited validity data available on existing measures, the authors surveyed a convenience sample of 55 emergency shelters, transitional housing programs, and housing programs serving families. The researchers rated the strength of assessment protocols (strong, adequate, deficient) across eight domains deemed important to supporting homeless families, based on their review of the literature. Across the domains, no protocol was judged to be strong, and only 4 of 55 (7%) were judged to be adequate.

Of the 93% of the assessments deemed deficient, most were deficient in multiple categories. The vast majority of protocols failed to address child development and parent functioning, and 96% did not include validated screening instruments.

This survey provides a loud wake-up call for responsive assessments of children and parents at entry into shelter. Without such baseline measures, services can't be matched to needs, and any objective determination of the effects of housing and services on well-being is impossible. The implications are clear: effective, tools and strategies for triage, screening, and assessment are critical to preventing the descent into homelessness, building family-centered strategies to shore up families once identified, and informing the field through ongoing data collection intended to meaningfully inform policy and practice.

Parent and Child Functioning: Where Do We Concentrate Effort?

The second study in this issue, by Herbers, Cutuli, Kolarova, Albu, and Sparks, also addresses families in emergency housing, engaging comprehensive, ongoing assessment. Studying a small sample ($N = 19$) of children and their parents (all single mothers), the researchers examined child and parent variables early in shelter stay and again 1 month later. Like other studies, they identified high rates of post-traumatic stress (PTS) and internalizing and externalizing behaviors among children. Perhaps the most interesting finding is that parents who experienced high distress underreported their children's traumatic stress symptoms. Whereas mothers' subjective ratings of PTS declined across time, children's did not. Parental warmth was not associated with child PTS or depression and children with higher executive function at entry showed higher internalizing symptoms later. We should note that this sample was restricted to children ages 8–11 years, significantly older than the typical age of children in family shelters. Nevertheless, thc findings raise issues for the field as to who should serve as respondent (child, parent, and/or provider, especially for younger children) and the need to incorporate multiple perspectives in the assessment of children engaged in homeless services. Additionally, more work is needed to understand the circumstances under which parents experiencing chronic, high levels of adversity are most attuned to child needs. Herbers et al.'s findings may be unsurprising given the emerging knowledge base about the effects of adverse childhood events (ACEs study, e.g., Dong et al., 2005) and the longstanding impact of toxic stress (Shonkoff et al., 2012); at the same time, they underscore the need to tailor existing research-supported interventions to the unique needs and assets of families experiencing or at risk for homelessness.

Engagement in Parenting Interventions: The Story Is in the Subgroups

Holtrop, Piehler, Gewirtz, and August also focus on parenting as a mediator of child adaptation among families who experiencing homelessness. The authors propose that the story is in the subgroups, that is, they concentrate on learning which subgroups of children and families benefit the most from parenting interventions. The "what works, for whom?" question isn't asked nearly as frequently as it should be. Some studies have found that higher risk families have more "room for improvement," whereas others have found them less likely to engage in (and benefit from) intervention. In this 2-year, cluster-randomized trial of the intensive Early Risers intervention, Holtrop et al. assessed competencies for 223 children of 137 single parents (98.5% female) who had previously experienced homelessness and were in stable housing with supportive services. About a third of the children had open child welfare cases at baseline. Interestingly, high distress families (with higher levels of parent depression and child behavior problems at baseline) showed greater improvements in observed parenting (e.g., reductions in use of ineffective discipline). The Early Risers approach is consistent with other efforts we have seen to stabilize the family first and then move to an intervention when the family is more ready to benefit from supports, lessons, and parenting techniques (e.g., Cunningham et al., 2014). The findings provide evidence for the effectiveness of housing as a platform for an array of interventions. We anticipate additional evidence as results emerge from five federally supported housing and child welfare demonstrations (USDHHS, 2012) and the Family Options Study (e.g., Gubits et al., 2015).

Community Collaboration in Support of Child Well-Being

Haskett, Tisdale, and Leonard Clay (this issue) report on a multi-tiered project and the role of community collaborations in promoting positive developmental and mental health outcomes for children who have experienced homelessness. The authors describe concerns about service gaps that occur when supports for homeless families are fragmented across multiple systems (e.g., housing, education, mental health) and present details of an elaborate effort to address interagency collaboration through the development of Community Action Targeting Children who are Homeless (CATCH), with a vision for a coordinated system of care. Project CATCH is funded through a blend of public and private resources, which is an interesting trend in the field. Haskett et al. are interested in systems-level changes (e.g., Foster-Fishman, Berkowitz, Lounsbury, Jacobson, & Allen, 2001) that might occur when shared goals lead to more coordinated and effective services for children who have experienced homelessness. In this case, the coordination focused on one North Carolina county and 11 housing agencies. The focus on a single county does raise the question of coordination across geographic borders as homeless or unstably housed families cross those boundaries.

The authors present a blend of qualitative and quantitative findings on collaborative meetings for community partners, trauma-informed care and support for shelter staff, several different types of "positive parenting" interventions for parents of young children, and—echoing other studies in this issue—the importance of developmental and mental health screenings for children experiencing homelessness. Overall, the coordinated and sustained efforts to bring partner agencies together to improve services for children are noteworthy. Mixed method approaches are well suited to the continuous feedback loop of engagement and improvement with community partners. Haskett et al.'s findings related to the effectiveness of parenting interventions, which varied greatly by model, dosage, delivery system, and measurement, are harder to interpret. The array of intervention approaches speaks to the complexity of service needs, program models, coordination across agencies, funding streams, data systems, and local decision-makers—and the need for ecological perspectives as collaborations form and evolve.

Haskett et al. conclude that intensive collaboration between housing and family-serving agencies is "feasible and valuable." Based on our own work, we agree and can also identify with lessons learned with respect to the challenges of coordination, the importance of having staff dedicated to the work (as a core role), and the need for near-constant messaging and retraining efforts, given high staff turnover rates in shelter and other service systems. If we are to replicate useful models, research needs to address the specific ingredients that promote collaboration, result in well-articulated practices for which implementation fidelity can be measured, and examine the role of leadership in convening and sustaining cross-systems collaboration.

Access to Early Childhood Services

In the final study, Perlman, Shaw, Kieffer, Whitney, and Bires share findings from an integrative mixed methods study, combining results from a quantitative National Association for the Education of Homeless Children and Youth (NAEHCY) survey of 970 professionals and Cloudburst Consulting Group's qualitative interviews with parents in 28 households who had participated in HUD's Family Options Study (e.g., Gubits et al., 2015). A majority of children entering emergency or transitional housing shelters are under the age of five, and these young children are also within the demographic group least likely to be stably housed. Given the literature on the impact of experiencing homelessness and/or housing instability on a host of educational outcomes during these early years (e.g., Fantuzzo, LeBoeuf, Chen, Rouse, & Culhane, 2012; Leventhal & Newman, 2010), the authors argue for better access to early childhood services for this vulnerable population.

McKinney-Vento
The McKinney-Vento Homeless Education Assistance Improvements Act of 2001, Subtitle B of title VII (42U.S.C. 11431 et seq.; http://www2.ed.gov/policy/elsec/leg/esea02/pg116.html) provides for "education for homeless children and youths." This legislation is widely credited for increasing dramatically the attention given to the educational needs of homeless children and youth. As the language below suggests, schools are required to track and report on the presence of homeless youth as well as the school's responsiveness to their needs. Of course, McKinney-Vento does not require schools to track or intervene in the case of housing instability (mobility), which is associated with reduced educational and social attainment (Fantuzzo et al., 2012), both in combination with episodes of homelessness and in of itself.
(1) Each State educational agency shall ensure that each child of a homeless individual and each homeless youth has equal access to the same free, appropriate public education, including a public preschool education, as provided to other children and youths.
(2) In any State that has a compulsory residency requirement as a component of the State's compulsory school attendance laws or other laws, regulations, practices, or policies that may act as a barrier to the enrollment, attendance, or success in school of homeless children and youths, the State will review and undertake steps to revise such laws, regulations, practices, or policies to ensure that homeless children and youths are afforded the same free, appropriate public education as provided to other children and youths.
(3) Homelessness alone is not sufficient reason to separate students from the mainstream school environment.
(4) Homeless children and youths should have access to the education and other services that such children and youths need to ensure that such children and youths have an opportunity to meet the same challenging State student academic achievement standards to which all students are held.

The Perlman et al. study revealed that families were often unaware of services and early childhood programs, and programs (with few incentives to investigate) were often unaware of the families in need. Systematic barriers included transportation availability and cost. In many instances, programs (e.g., Head Start and Title I preschools) existed in the community but had such long waiting lists that they were effectively unavailable. The kind of collaboration and communication advocated by Haskett et al. (this issue) seemed mostly absent, as shelters and families often lacked knowledge about how to access early childhood services. Perlman et al. emphasize the importance of the McKinney-Vento Homeless Assistance Act for the improvement of homeless students' access to and success in public schools. They call for its extension to cover federally funded early care and education programs, too. Perhaps schools could be further leveraged to other services through the McKinney-Vento liaisons; re-envisioning the roles of schools may be part of a more comprehensive strategy to meet the complex needs of unstably housed and homeless families. Although McKinney-Vento has brought attention and a legal tool to aid students, many would argue that limited funding and enforcement hamper its impact. Disincentives to serve homeless children (e.g., costs associated with transportation, special services) pose barriers within school districts. Training, funding, and systems-level changes that reward districts for the successful education of homeless children need attention. Nonetheless, the authors' main point about the need to extend similar protections to early care and education programs is valid.

Policy Resources and Next Steps

In 2010, the USICH presented the *Opening Doors* plan to prevent and end family homelessness by 2020. Problems as complex as family homelessness in America rarely respond to unidimensional solutions. The plan calls for coordinated, sustainable, cross-systems partnerships such as those articulated by Haskett et al. (this issue). Public–private partnerships provide excellent opportunities for learning (e.g., demonstrations of effectiveness), and we do wonder about the mid- to long-term implications: who is "responsible" for maintaining collaborative partnerships and evaluating "success" over the long term? Efforts must be made to address the so-called wrong pocket problem in which money spent by one agency (e.g., early childhood screening and services) on effective prevention/intervention that saves money for a second agency (e.g., costs of shelter or special education) isn't credited to the first agency. In our experience, states and localities (given the need to produce balanced budgets) may be more responsive to this issue than has been the U.S. federal government to date; that is, federal policy around housing (in particular, families and youth) is fragmented and does not entail a single system, rather, comprises separate programs and funding streams that do not form a coherent set of practices.

Policy and Practice Websites of Note

- Opening Doors, the U.S. Interagency Council on Homelessness (http://usich.gov/opening_doors/)
- The National Center on Family Homelessness (http://www.familyhomelessness.org) ranks states based on: (1) extent of child homelessness; (2) child well-being; (3) risk for child homelessness; and (4) state policy and planning efforts.
- The Administration for Children and Family, U.S. Department of Health and Human Services, published a 2016 report on "Early childhood homelessness in the United States: 50-state profile" (https://www.acf.hhs.gov/sites/default/files/ecd/homelessness_profile_package_with_blanks_for_printing_508.pdf).
- The National Center for Housing and Child Welfare (http://www.nchcw.org/advocacy-and-policy.html) provides excellent federal policy updates, with a focus on families involved in child welfare.
- The National Association for the Education of Homeless Children and Youth (NAEHCY) hosts an annual conference and provides policy-related technical assistance to promote educational excellence for students experiencing homelessness (http://www.naehcy.org/).
- The National Center for Homeless Education (NCHE; http://center.serve.org/nche/index.php) is the U.S. Department of Education's information and technical assistance center for the federal Education for Homeless Children and Youth (EHCY) Program. The NCHE website includes issue and practice briefs, online training resources, legislation and policy information, and links to national, state, and local resources.
- An example of a site that highlights science-based practices for working with children and families is InfoAboutKids (http://infoaboutkids.org), a collaboration across seven divisions (including Division 37) of the American Psychological Association.

The policy implications are clear: funding for service models and evaluation alike, if not longitudinal in reach, will fail to inform long-term solutions to family homelessness. The fragmented nature of family policymaking and the siloed nature of federal and state budgeting pose significant challenges to sustainability and replicability. Election cycles and leadership changes complicate community and systems efforts by imposing artificial transitions. By virtue of their relatively longitudinal and enduring approach to resource and practice, private–public partnerships may be uniquely poised to sustain cross-systems collaborative efforts.

The studies in this issue describe homeless children and families' characteristics and co-occurring risk factors, which become important as we consider how they enter into the various systems that attempt to address their needs. Clearly, coordinated entry in each Continuum of Care must include improved assessment of child and parent needs and competencies (DeCandia et al., this issue; Herbers et al., this issue). There is evidence that long-term housing supports are important to stabilize homeless families (e.g., Gubits et al., 2015), but, as DeCandia et al. suggest, we must also study and understand the quality and effectiveness of supportive services that may be delivered once the basic need of housing is met. Further, triage and assessment need to be embedded across family-serving systems and institutions (child care, education, housing, health, child welfare) if we are to realize the *Opening Doors* objective of prevention and swift intervention tailored to family assets and needs. The results of the small but rigorous study by Holtrop et al. (this issue) contribute to our understanding of who may best respond to specific interventions and prompt new queries about matching services and intensity to family needs. The viability of future policies and programs depends on the field's capacity to compose an evidence-informed, cost-effective continuum of prevention and intervention services.

Most of the studies in this issue (and elsewhere) focus on single parent families headed by women with young children. Certainly, shelters are not contexts of choosing for families; the optimal context is a permanent, safe home in a desired community, starting early in life. The evidence presented here, and the knowledge base on the long-term impact of quality early childhood programs, highlights the dramatic need for increased access to early care and education services for young children experiencing homelessness or housing instability (Perlman et al., this issue). Provisions in the reauthorized Child Care Development Block Grant (CCDBG) of 2014 have incorporated McKinney-Vento concepts into the policies of the Individuals with Disabilities Education Act (IDEA) and Head Start. Depending on funding levels and implementation, the CCDBG may provide additional resources to homeless providers to help their clients tap early childhood resources. Haskett et al. (this issue) note that the Improving Head Start for School Readiness Act of 2007 mandated the prioritization of young children (birth to five) experiencing homelessness. Waitlists still persist, however, reminding us of the need for appropriations of resources to follow mandates. There may be additional barriers to family participation in Head Start for unstably housed and homeless families, including the place-based nature of eligibility and access (among other factors) to Head Start and the realities that families face in transporting children to programs. Given the disproportionate number of families with infants who are homeless, Early Start and related infant care programs may provide critical opportunities to intervene with families at risk for homelessness. Even before that, newborn services and pediatric medical home models (e.g., Project DULCE: Developmental Understanding & Legal Collaboration for Everyone; Sege et al., 2015) provide early opportunities to query families about housing status and to connect them with critical supports.

The families served in shelters and other housing services have limited education and work histories, are disproportionately African American or Hispanic, and are more likely than their stably housed low income counterparts to experience domestic violence, behavioral health concerns, and child welfare involvement. Data from the National Survey of Child and Adolescent Well-Being reveal that inadequate housing frequently contributed to removal from home among children in child welfare-involved families (Fowler et al., 2013). The Family Unification Program (FUP) provides Housing Choice Vouchers to families for whom the lack of adequate housing is a risk factor for out-of-home placement or delay in family. One policy initiative of note is a bill introduced in the U.S. Senate (S.1964; Family Stability and Kinship Care Act of 2015) would amend Part E (Foster Care and Adoption Assistance) of Title IV of the Social Security Act to give states added flexibility to fund preventive services (including housing supports) to stabilize families and to prevent child removal and placement in foster care. As we write this, the Bill has been read and referred to the Committee on Finance.

Empirical understanding of these co-occurring risks must inform policy, practice, and studies that seek to understand what works in preventing family homelessness, coordinating entry and housing and support systems, and tracking outcomes across a variety of administrative systems. Likewise, the field needs to better understand the sources of resilience that enable a subset of vulnerable children, families, and youth to adjust and (yes) thrive, in spite of adversity.

Key Steps to Ending Family Homelessness: Bassuk Center
The Bassuk Center on Homeless and Vulnerable Children and Youth (BassukCenter.org) is an important new resource for the analysis of federal policy on family homelessness. In their report on "Services matter: How housing and services can end family homelessness" (Bassuk, DeCandia, & Richard, 2015), the Center recommends eight (interrelated) components that must be part of the response. These eight recommendations are well supported by the articles in this volume. According to the report, agencies and service systems must:
1) Provide permanent affordable housing in the community
2) Support economic self-sufficiency
3) Assess all family members
4) Address trauma-related issues
5) Treat depression in mothers
6) Minimize family separations
7) Provide parenting supports
8) Address children's needs

In Connecticut, an interagency working group has proposed a plan that aligns well with these recommendations. Spanning the Office of Early Childhood, Department of Social Services, Department of Housing, and Department of Children and Families, among other agencies and partners, the group seeks to align definitions of child, youth, and family homelessness, coordinate data and services, and target funding. In particular, the plan is for more access to coordinated health care, child care and early education (e.g., child care subsidies), and housing supports (e.g., homeless families as a priority in the HUD administrative plan). As we write this, the CT Office of Early Childhood contemplates concrete steps (screening for family risks and assets) to insure that severe housing instability and homelessness among families with young children are identified as early as possible so as to maximize the window of time available to shore up families, ultimately to the benefit and well-being of children.

Our review of the articles in this issue leaves us feeling simultaneously encouraged and challenged. In the table below, we summarize the collective wisdom of the scholars whose work appears in this brief—and beyond—by offering a set of observations and aspirations for the field in the form of policy and practice recommendations. Our nation's commitment to the well-being of children and families is hearteningly evident within *Opening Doors*. The research contained here offers a helpful roadmap for practice and underscores the need for continuing knowledge development. Yet we face clear resource gaps as we contemplate next steps; for example, if we have effective means to screen and triage families with housing vulnerability and develop the workforce capacity to enact these methods with sensitivity, but lack the requisite community resources to which families can be referred, we have not created viable solutions. The desired outcome of an attuned, family-centered screening and assessment process is *not* a waitlist for services. Further, we cannot end homelessness without preventing it. These observations indeed suggest a concerted, data-informed perspective on program design coupled with developmental evaluation approaches (Gamble, 2008) that enable providers to match levels of support with family typologies and to understand the impact of their work. We call on scholars and practitioners to utilize the resources and lessons from the empirical articles in this issue of *Advances in Child and Family Policy and Practice* to move forward with practices, policies, and research that will improve the lives of children, youth, and families who experience or are at risk for homelessness. We've come a long way, and we have a long way to go.

Policy Implications and Recommendations
Taken together, the articles in this issue, combined with the growing body of knowledge about the effects of frank homelessness and housing instability, and the four capacities outlined in *Opening Doors*, suggest the need for additional knowledge development and we provide some suggestions for future research. In the meantime, policy development, program design, and related work necessarily continues under the careful leadership of highly skilled implementers and with the guidance of the accumulated body of knowledge.
Policy
• We are encouraged by the cross-systems emphasis of recent legislative efforts and hope this continues. For example, the Family Unification Modernization and Improvement Act of 2015 was recently introduced to Congress. The Act, if passed, would enable incentives for the use of evidence-based practices and promote interagency coordination and accountability.

(continued)

• Additionally, we believe that future policy initiatives can reflect the growing awareness that ending homelessness requires preventing it. This is the bold approach taken by the *Opening Doors* initiative, and realizing it requires an integrated approach that enables the articulation of an array of family assets and needs with programmatic approaches and components. Perlman and colleagues (this issue) find that, among children, infants are most likely to be identified as homeless. Whereas this finding reminds us of the peril of longstanding neurocognitive effects of homelessness and trauma, it can be recast as an opportunity for prevention and early intervention.
Program Design, Evaluation, and Research
• The phenomena of family housing instability and homelessness are associated with limited health, social, behavioral, and academic progress among children and youth. Ecological approaches to shoring up vulnerable families (e.g., match the program intensity to family need) have important potential. Future programmatic efforts may be more efficient and effective if they capitalize on an understanding of family needs in order to provide a sufficient "dosage" of services and promote the "right amount" of family engagement to produce sustainable change.
• Undoubtedly, the randomized trials that are underway will produce actionable information; at the same time, variations in the composition of systems and services within and across states and regions necessarily limits the extent to which findings can inform the field. It is critical that those findings not be interpreted as simple judgments of success or failure; instead, they can inform future developmental evaluations that apply lessons learned.

References

Bassuk, E. L., DeCandia, C. J., & Richard, M. K. (2015). *Services matter: How housing and services can end family homelessness*. Needham, MA: The Bassuk Center on Homeless and Vulnerable Children and Youth. Retrieved from http://www.bassukcenter.org/wp-content/uploads/2015/11/Services-Matter.pdf

Bassuk, E. L., DeCandia, C. J., Tsertsvadze, A., & Richard, M. K. (2014). The effectiveness of housing interventions and housing and service interventions on ending family homelessness: A systematic review. *American Journal of Orthopsychiatry*, *84*, 457–474. doi:10.1037/ort0000020.

Cunningham, M. K., Pergamit, M., McDaniel, M., Gearing, M., Zhang, S., & Howell, B. (2014). *Supportive housing for high-need families in the child welfare system*. Retrieved from http://www.urban.org/UploadedPDF/2000010-Supportive-Housing-for-High-Need-Families-in-the-Child-Welfare-System.pdf?RSSFeed=Urban.xml

Dong, M., Anda, R. F., Felitti, V. J., Williamson, D. F., Dube, S. R., Brown, D. W., & Giles, W. H. (2005). Childhood residential mobility and multiple health risks during adolescence and adulthood: The hidden role of adverse childhood experiences. *Archives of Pediatrics & Adolescent Medicine*, *159*(12), 1104–1110. doi:10.1001/archpedi.159.12.1104.

Fantuzzo, J. W., LeBoeuf, W. A., Chen, C.-C., Rouse, H. L., & Culhane, D. P. (2012). The unique and combined effects of homelessness and school mobility on the educational outcomes of young children. *Educational Researcher*, *41*, 393–402. doi:10.3102/0013189X12468210.

Farrell, A. F., Britner, P. A., Guzzardo, M., & Goodrich, S. (2010). Supportive housing for families in child welfare: Client characteristics and their outcomes at discharge. *Children and Youth Services Review*, *32*, 145–154. doi:10.1016/j.childyouth.2009.06.012.

Foster-Fishman, P. G., Berkowitz, S. L., Lounsbury, D. W., Jacobson, S., & Allen, N. A. (2001). Building collaborative capacity in community coalitions: A review and integrative framework. *American Journal of Community Psychology*, *29*, 241–261. doi:10.1023/A:1010378613583.

Fowler, P. J., Henry, D. B., Schoeny, M., Landsverk, J., Chavira, D., & Taylor, J. J. (2013). Inadequate housing among families under investigation for child abuse and neglect: Prevalence from a national probability sample. *American Journal of Community Psychology, 52*, 106–114. doi:10.1007/s10464-013-9580-8.

Gamble, J. A. (2008). *A developmental evaluation primer*. Montreal: JW McConnell Family Foundation.

Grant, R., Gracy, D., Goldsmith, G., Shapiro, A., & Redlener, I. E. (2013). Twenty-five years of child and family homelessness: Where are we now? *American Journal of Public Health, 103* (S2), e1–e10. doi:10.2105/AJPH.2013.301618.

Gubits, D., Shinn, M., Bell, S., Wood, M., Dastrup, S., Solari, C. D., … McInnis, D. (2015). *Family options study: Short-term impacts of housing and services interventions for homeless families*. Washington, DC: U.S. Department of Housing and Urban Development, Office of Policy Development and Research.

Leventhal, T., & Newman, S. (2010). Housing and child development. *Children and Youth Services Review, 32*(9), 1165–1174. doi:10.1016/j.childyouth.2010.03.008.

Sege, R., Preer, G., Morton, S. J., Cabral, H., Morakinyo, O., Lee, V., … Kaplan-Sanoff, M. (2015). Medical-legal strategies to improve infant health care: A randomized trial. *Pediatrics, 136*(1), 97–106. doi:10.1542/peds.2014-2955.

Shonkoff, J. P., Garner, A. S., the Committee on Psychosocial Aspects of Child and Family Health, & Committee on Early Childhood, Adoption, and Dependent Care, and Section on Developmental and Behavioral Pediatrics (2012). The lifelong effects of early childhood adversity and toxic stress. *Pediatrics, 129*(1), e232–e246. doi:10.1542/peds.2011-2663.

U.S. Department of Health and Human Services. (2012). *Partnerships to demonstrate the effectiveness of supportive housing for families in the child welfare system*. Retrieved from http://www.acf.hhs.gov/hhsgrantsforecast/index.cfm?switch=grant.view&gff_grants_forecastInfoID=38683

U.S. Interagency Council on Homelessness (2015). *Opening doors: Federal strategic plan to end homelessness*. Washington, DC: U.S. Interagency Council on Homelessness.

Index

M.E. Haskett (ed.), *Child and Family Well-Being and Homelessness*,
SpringerBriefs in Psychology, DOI 10.1007/978-3-319-50886-3

The manufacturer's authorised representative in the EU is Springer Nature Customer Service Centre GmbH, Europaplatz 3, 69115 Heidelberg, Germany. If you have any concerns regarding our products, please contact ProductSafety@springernature.com

Printed and bound by CPI Group (UK) Ltd, Croydon, CR0 4YY
30/09/2026
02225468-0015